While caring for newborns as a family physician, I'm often asked about infant development. Parental concerns are frequently followed by different variations of the same question: "Is my baby's behavior normal?" I'm convinced every new mom goes through this type of anxiety.

Ginny Cruz offers an indispensable resource to help alleviate those fears in her book, *The New Mom's Guide: Help and Hope for Baby's First Year.* As an experienced pediatric physical therapist, she presents sound guidance on important developmental milestones in small bites of information ideally geared for the new mother's harried schedule. But she also includes references with every chapter for a more in-depth study of the topic if so desired.

This guide is certainly an essential addition to every new mom's library as well as the perfect shower gift before the baby's anticipated arrival.

— Suzanne Montgomery, MD, FAAFP

As a speech-language pathologist, I wholeheartedly endorse Ginny Cruz's book. I have worked alongside her for nearly ten years. Her expertise as a physical therapist and her understanding of early childhood development shine through in this insightful, practical guide. The book offers a clear, compassionate approach to understanding and supporting developmental needs. Ginny's book is an invaluable resource for parents, educators, and professionals alike. This work is a must-read for anyone committed to fostering growth and love!

— Alita Fisher, M.S., CCC-SLP

As a pediatric occupational therapist for over forty-two years, I have worked with very few pediatric physical therapists as knowledgeable and skillful as Ginny Cruz. I've had the privilege of working directly with her in a clinical setting and have followed her career for thirty years. Her vast knowledge and expertise in infant motor and sensory development, so critical in the baby's first year, are outstanding. More importantly, her ability to teach parents and caregivers these concepts in a very practical way is a special gift. I am certain that whoever reads this book will gain greater confidence in understanding their baby's developmental needs throughout the first year of life.

— Laura Mitchell, OT (Retired)/ Certified in NDT, SI, and infant massage

Ginny Cruz has all the qualities you want in a teacher, coach, and mentor! Having worked with Ginny in Early Intervention for about a decade, I have learned so much from her and will forever be grateful for that! She was always there when I had a question, willing to teach and explain in simple terms while demonstrating hands-on when needed. When Ginny and I evaluated infants and toddlers for the Early Intervention program, she brought knowledge, kindness, compassion, support, and honesty to the table. She was always advocating for the babies and families, and she continues to do so!

— Jenelle Segno, B.A., ITDS

The New Mom's Guide

Help and Hope for Baby's First Year

Ginny Cruz, MPA, PT

Cover design and interior formatting by *Hannah Linder Designs*

Disclaimer

All information provided reflects general guidelines and general recommendations. It is not intended as specific medical advice for your child. If you have concerns about any aspect of your child's development, talk with their doctor. If your child is receiving therapy, please share this information with the therapist.

Contents

Section Two
Four To Six Months

Section Three
Seven To Nine Months

To my mom and grandmothers, who set the standard for love, devotion, and steadfast duty in the role of mother. There has never been a day I didn't reflect on and strive to follow your example.

To all mothers. May you seek guidance from those with wisdom to share. While each generation has a new twist, there's nothing new under the sun. All babies need love, guidance, boundaries, and patience.

Introduction

Looking for proven ways to help your baby successfully meet first-year milestones? Then this book is for you. It includes tips on how to play with your baby in ways that promote healthy development. The book also offers inspiration and humor to provide some levity and encouragement when you think you can't go on another second. Consulting this resource is an active way to show how much you love your baby.

When my husband and I took custody of our first adopted child, he came with the clothes on his back, blue-and-red sandals, and legal paperwork. No extra food or diapers, and most importantly, no instruction manual. Everything in my life up to that point had prepared me for the work world, but not for the job I now held—mother. I recognized this role was the most important one I'd ever had, and I didn't want to mess it up. You may feel that way too.

In my former role as a pediatric physical therapist and early intervention specialist, I spoke with mothers who felt as overwhelmed as I did many years ago. I heard their fears and recalled my own. *How do I help my baby calm down? Is my child okay? What am I doing wrong?* Unfortunately, motherhood often feels like you're going from one problem to another, forced to figure it out alone.

The New Mom's Guide: Help and Hope for Baby's First Year is my gift to you. It's the book I wish I'd had at the beginning of my own motherhood journey. My prayer is that the stories comfort you, make you laugh, and help your baby stay on track.

You may feel alone on the motherhood trail, but you aren't. *The New Mom's Guide* is my way of coming alongside you and scattering crumbs along the path to guide your steps.

Section One

Birth to Three Months

Chapter 1

Love at First Sight

A baby is born with a need to be loved
—and never outgrows it.[1]

I saw my oldest child for the first time in a photograph, but it wasn't a sonogram. My husband and I were adopting, and the agency gave us a thick packet of information, which contained many pages detailing his birth information, physical characteristics, and health information. But I only wanted to study that photograph. His radiant smile and button-brown eyes captivated me. He was *the one for us.*

Although I never gave birth, many mothers tell me it was love at first sight for them in the delivery room. Most describe an overwhelming sense of love for their baby. If you didn't feel that way, I hope your love for your baby has grown.

Circumstances surrounding a child's birth can be difficult. But look at the quote above again. Every baby needs love. Two of the best ways to love your baby are holding them and paying attention to them.

Your baby loves your smell, heartbeat, and voice. When your baby sees and touches you, they experience love at first sight also. During these intimate moments with your baby, you can nurture their development in numerous ways. Some of the following suggestions may seem simple, but they have proven effective for most babies.

Ways to Encourage Your Baby's Development:

- Convey a tactile sense of safety. Your newborn relies on touch and smell to detect your presence. Holding your baby conveys safety, love, and protection.
- Do Kangaroo Care or skin-to-skin contact. Place your diapered baby against your chest with skin touching skin. Dads can do this too. While often used with premature babies, Kangaroo Care works with all babies. Skin-to-skin contact helps your baby stop crying, to gain weight, and to regulate vital functions, such as maintaining body temperature, heartbeat, and breathing rate. Gaining weight and maintaining body temperature will give your baby the energy to grow stronger and stay awake to play.

Things to Remember:

Your eyes remind me of:

____.

I can't get enough of your:

____.

Chapter 2

First Breath

Your first breath took ours away.[1]

What did you feel when you heard your baby's first cry? Did you wonder if your baby was in pain? Were you relieved both of you were still alive?

When your baby first cries after birth, they breathe oxygen into their lungs. But did you know your baby's circulatory and respiratory systems must rapidly switch from functioning in the amniotic fluid of the womb to thriving outside in the air? Amazing, right? Premature babies may not be ready to make this switcheroo, which accounts for many preemies struggling to breathe.

Full-term babies arrive wired for an immediate conversion to breathing air so they can survive in their new environment. Mothers, on the other hand, usually need more time to figure out how to care for their baby.

Your doctor didn't hand you an owner's manual after your baby's birth. Motherhood is an on-the-job training program that will require every ounce of your strength and willpower on most days. But from that first moment through every future one, you will do your best.

Live moment by moment, take deep breaths, and learn to be okay with feeling unprepared. Chaos comes with the job. But you may soon agree with many other moms that motherhood is the best and most challenging job ever.

Ways to Encourage Your Baby's Development:

- Cuddle your baby and inhale the sweet scent from their head.
- Remind yourself to close your eyes and take a few deep breaths throughout the day. Tell yourself, "I'm doing okay." No one else may tell you, so tell yourself.

Things to Remember:

Your APGAR scores at birth were

____.

My labor lasted ______ hours.

Chapter 3

What's in a Name?

We call her Sexy Pants.[1]

Our evaluation team huddled in a small examination room, assessing the development of an on-the-move, easily distractible toddler. The child didn't respond when we called her name, which was long and difficult to pronounce. After a few attempts, the speech pathologist asked the child's mother, "Do you have a nickname for her?" The mom giggled, then replied, "We call her Sexy Pants."

The speech therapist called out, "Come here, Sexy Pants!" The child turned around and looked at us. She didn't come, but she demonstrated she knew and responded to the name Sexy Pants.

Naming a child can be tricky. Do you go with a family name, one of someone you love and admire, a famous person, or one you create? I'm old-fashioned, so I prefer names that have stood the test of time and have historical significance. To me, trendy choices carry minimal history. On the other hand, maybe you love your child's given name but now use a pet name anyway. A nickname is fine, but may this true story gently remind you that your baby's pet name may not sound as cute when spoken by strangers.

What's in a Name?

I once treated a child nicknamed Biscuit. That's a story for another day.

Ways to Encourage Your Baby's Development:

- Make up songs that include your baby's name, which will make them feel special.
- Address your baby by their name. For example, "(Baby's name), do you want to eat?" This teaches your baby to recognize their name and enlarges their vocabulary.

Things to Remember:

Your nickname or pet name is

______________________________________.

Names we almost selected for you were

______________________________.

Chapter 4

Looks Like

It's the universal mom rant: We put in the work, but Dad gets the genetic credit.[1]

Whom does your baby favor? I'm sure you've talked about that and reached some conclusions. Maybe your mother said, "He's got your eyes," or you said, "I think he has his father's nose." From the first moment you saw your child, you searched for familiar characteristics. Even parents of adopted children see uncanny resemblances. My husband and I continue to be amazed at the similarities we discover in our two adopted sons.

Many moms I've helped over my years in pediatric physical therapy have shared their frustration that their baby's first word is dada. Unfortunately, all mothers seem to share this sentiment. We resent that daddy gets called first when we have done so much work. Maybe that's meant to remind us that our role as mother—while vital—is serving the needs of others. And on those days we feel forgotten and unappreciated, we may slip into feeling sorry for ourselves. If this resonates with you, you aren't alone. Yes, dada is often the first word your baby says, but never fear—once they learn to say mama, you'll wish they called dada every time they need something.

Ways to Encourage Your Baby's Development:

- Make funny faces as you look at each other. Sticking out your tongue or blowing kisses teaches your baby to imitate actions. These activities also increase social and emotional connections.
- Delegate some baby care tasks to dad. Your child develops critical social skills by playing and interacting with others.

Things to Remember:

You look like your daddy in the following ways:

____.

You love it when your dad

____.

Chapter 5

Your Baby's Skin

A baby's vision is still developing after birth, so they recognize people and places by their scent. That means when you hold your baby or enter their room, they may recognize you not by how you look, but how you smell.[1]

Do you love to cuddle your baby and smell their skin? Many mothers have told me they love that new-baby smell. Here's another sweet nugget of information—your baby knows and loves how *your* skin smells. Yes, they know it's you.

The sense of smell is one of the first senses your baby develops in utero. From birth, your baby bonds with your scent and knows you by how you smell, not by how you look. Lots of snuggling and cuddling cements strong memories and develops love and trust between you and your child. So, snuggle and cuddle. Show your baby that your touch is safe and gentle, and they'll associate those memories with your scent. You smell like love and safety, and that's what you want your little one to know about you. You are their safe place.

WAYS TO ENCOURAGE YOUR BABY'S DEVELOPMENT:

- Snuggle and sway your baby gently. These movements and touches convey comfort and safety.
- Sing the song "I Love You, You Love Me" over your baby or another one that emphasizes your love.

THINGS TO REMEMBER:

One of my favorite scents from my childhood was

____.

You seem to love the smell of

____.

Chapter 6

Mother's Milk

Breast milk is the best source of nutrition for most babies.[1]

Your body was designed to birth, nourish, and nurture your baby. So, you might think this design would work well for all moms. But it doesn't. Breastfeeding can be difficult for many mothers and babies. When breastfeeding is challenging, many moms become discouraged and feel as if they're not "good enough."

Yes, breast milk is the best food for most babies. But in some situations, your baby may struggle to drink your milk. Some babies can't latch; others get tired and can't take in enough milk to gain weight. Seek help from their doctor in these cases. Some mothers feed breast milk through a bottle or go straight to formula. Whichever you choose, your baby's health is the most important consideration—not what others think.

No matter your choice, all mothers battle feelings of not being "good enough" in one way or another.

Moms can also struggle with feeding themselves during the early months of motherhood. But feeding your body may not be the main problem; it may be lack of nourishment for your spirit. I recommend reading the Bible, praying for strength and guidance, and talking about your struggles with good friends. These are effective ways to feed your spirit. Don't neglect your own needs during this time in your baby's life. Both of you need physical and emotional sustenance.

Ways to Encourage Your Baby's Development:

- Feed your baby the best milk you can in whatever way you can. Don't allow guilt or other people's opinions to steal your joy.
- Switch sides (right and left) as you feed your baby. Changing sides occurs naturally with breastfeeding but not with bottle feeds. Switching sides allows your baby to strengthen their mouth and neck muscles more thoroughly.

Things to Remember:

When it came to breastfeeding, you

____.

Do you prefer breastmilk or formula?_________________.

If formula, your favorite brand is___________________.

Chapter 7

Overwhelmed

Being a mother is discovering strengths you didn't know you had and dealing with fears you never knew existed.[1]

He wouldn't stop crying no matter what we did. Our first son was sixteen months old when we adopted him, and we spent our first night together in a hotel room in Manila, Philippines. That evening I felt overwhelmed by the many unknowns I faced with this new baby. I had no book, no previous experience, and no place to find the answers. Curled up on the cold bathroom floor, I fought nausea and stomach cramps. My mind raced with questions: *How are we going to survive flying sixteen hours on a plane back to the United States if he's going to scream like this? How will I handle traveling with a new child? What if we can't get back home?*

Those fears and others engulfed me that first night with our newly adopted son. Maybe you've felt something similar. If so, you aren't alone. According to the American Pregnancy Association, 70–80 percent of all new mothers experience some negative feelings or mood swings after giving birth.[2] Adoptive moms can also have mood swings.

During those paralyzing days of fear on the long trip back to the United States and through the early days of adjustment to our new lives, I rediscovered prayer. You bet I called out to God while I sat on that bathroom floor. Every time I felt overwhelmed with fear, I cried out to Him and even when I had no words, He calmed my concerns. Looking back, I realize my worries were baseless.

Motherhood is stressful. Talk to someone you trust when you become anxious. Be humble enough to admit you're overwhelmed. I talked to God and those I trusted with my deepest insecurities. Every mother is learning on the job even though she may project the image of perfection. Most experienced moms will admit they don't know how they did it all, but they did. You will too. You have strengths you haven't tapped into yet.

Ways to Encourage Your Baby's Development:

- When you feel overwhelmed, call a trusted friend or meet with your pastor. If you need mental health assistance, get it. Your baby needs you to be healthy and present.
- Take walks with your baby. Walking releases hormones that calm your mind. The motion also calms your baby.

Things to Remember:

You won't stop crying unless I

____.

You're so cute when I dress you in

____.

Chapter 8

Tongue-Tied

Tongue-tie is a hereditary medical condition that affects 2 to 4 percent of infants, and in some cases can impact the ability to breastfeed successfully.[1]

Many new moms have never heard of tongue-ties or lip ties. Maybe you thought your tongue was tied when you became flustered during a speech and couldn't speak. "Did you get tongue-tied?" your friend may ask, because this is an everyday slang use of the term. No, your tongue was not tied. You just got a dry mouth and became anxious. But tongue-ties and lip ties are actual medical conditions.

A tongue-tie is a malformation that restricts the movement of the tongue and can cause a speech impediment. A lip tie is a malformation that restricts the movement of the lips. There are varying levels of severity, and some babies experience both tongue and lip ties.

This fairly common condition is often missed in all the activities during and immediately after birth until latching and feeding issues arise. Some doctors recommend doing nothing and letting it take care of itself. Others will want to release the restriction surgically.

Common symptoms of tongue-tie in infants are:

Tongue-Tied

1. Does not latch well,
2. Chews more than sucks,
3. Fussy during feeding time,
4. Makes a clicking noise when feeding,
5. Always seems hungry, and
6. Feeds for a long time, takes a short break, and then feeds for another extended period.

Unless your baby isn't gaining weight, what to do about the tie is your decision. If your baby is exhausted by feeding and not growing properly, the tongue-tie may need to be fixed so your child can feed easily and gain weight.

Ways to Encourage Your Baby's Development:

- To check for tongue-tie, lay your baby down on their back facing you. Gently run your finger under their tongue. A normal tongue will allow for a smooth and uninterrupted swipe. However, your baby may have a tongue-tie if the tissue under the tongue feels short, firm, or excessively thick. Talk with your baby's doctor about your concerns.
- Encourage your baby to blow raspberries.

Things to Remember:

I love those sucking sounds you make while feeding.
I first thought about tongue-tie when you were ____months old.

Chapter 9

White Noise

Pediatricians recommend that any white noise machines be placed at least seven feet away from your baby's crib and you should keep the volume on the machine below the maximum setting.[1]

When my sons were babies, I installed air cleaners in their rooms. The steady hum of the fan created white noise that blocked out other sounds. As a result, they slept better, and the constant hum in the background calmed them and helped quiet their overactive minds and bodies.

Now that they're grown, they still use an air cleaner in the bedroom because they love that white noise. But since they've always slept on camping or trips without the noise, I don't believe they're addicted to it, which is one of the drawbacks of using it.

I also love certain noises, such as a fan running or a steady rain, and I've always slept better while hearing them. Do certain sounds help you sleep better? If your baby struggles with sleep, try a little white noise. Experiment with different types, such as soft rain or heart-beat sounds. Different children enjoy different sounds. But don't place the machine near the bed. Many of the sound machines on the market are too loud (higher than fifty decibels) and can, over the long term, harm your child's hearing.

Ways to Encourage Your Baby's Development:

- Darken the room to help your baby get deep rest.
- Take your doctor's advice and sleep when you can.

Things to Remember:

You sleep best with _____________________sounds.
I'm currently functioning on an average of ______hours of sleep.

Chapter 10

The Nose Knows

New research shows that women have more cells in the olfactory bulb—the area of the brain that is dedicated to sense of smell—than men.[1]

When I first held my newly adopted babies, my first action was to kiss and smell the tops of their heads. Kissing a baby's head must be instinctual.

Bonding with your baby includes knowing how they smell. Babies also learn the smell of their mothers. Both noses sense they belong together.

As the days and years advance, your mother's nose will encounter new smells. Some will be pleasant aromas—clean laundry, for example. Other ones, like soured milk and baby diarrhea, are gag-inducing. You know this already. If not, you will.

Scientific research shows women have more brain cells devoted to sensing and discriminating smells than men do. Of course, the extra focus must be related to our survival and our baby's well-being. Have you ever smelled something, like rank milk, and your husband replies, "It smells fine to me." As I said, mothers need a better sense of smell.

Yes, there will be awful odors, but there are also beautiful ones.

The Nose Knows

Lavender-scented clothes, birthday cake, and baby wipes will be familiar scents your mother's nose will adore. Of course, we all laugh about the dirty diapers and spit up, but those are minor inconveniences to endure as you enjoy the journey.

Ways to Encourage Your Baby's Development:

- Be cautious with introducing your baby to artificial scents, like perfumes or air fresheners, until you know if your baby is allergic to them.
- Label the names of smells for your baby. Say things like, "You smell like lavender" or "Do you smell the grass?"

Things to Remember:

The worst odor I ever smelled was

____.

I spend a lot of time doing laundry.

CHAPTER 11

TEARS

Sometime between 1 and 3 months of age is when most babies begin shedding real tears.[1]

While *you* may have shed a few tears since your baby arrived, your baby may not have shed a tear yet. You've probably cried tears of joy, exhaustion, or anger. And sometimes you don't even know why your eyes leak. Your baby has cried and even sobbed. But not until one to three months will real tears roll down your baby's cheeks.

When those first tears appear, your baby's crying may be more difficult to tolerate. Wet, salty tears glistening on those sweet baby cheeks will tug at your heartstrings even more.

Tears are salty because they contain electrolytes from the body and are a cleansing agent, much like sweat. Crying is as natural a body function as breathing. Since it comes with deep sadness or buried emotions, some have described tears as waves crashing on the shore. They bring a healing release of energy and renewal.

Your baby will often cry for no apparent reason. Most cries indicate hunger or discomfort. Remember, tears are your baby's only way to let you know they need something. Motherhood contains thousands of frustrating moments as you try to figure out what your baby needs so they'll stop crying. In those times, reflect on how many times you've cried and didn't know why. Maybe you just needed the emotional release, or maybe you wanted someone's attention. Babies are just like us. They don't always know what they need or want. Often they want to be held, comforted, and told, "I love you." Do you blame them?

WAYS TO ENCOURAGE YOUR BABY'S DEVELOPMENT:

- Respond to your baby's cries and do your best to meet those needs. Your consistent actions tell your baby you're trustworthy.
- Keep regular routines with your baby. Predictable patterns calm and project a stable environment. The more relaxed your baby is, the happier you'll be.

THINGS TO REMEMBER:

Things that usually calm your crying are

____.

Things that make me cry right now are

____.

Chapter 12

Sole Care

Each foot has over 200,000 nerve endings.[1]

Moms instinctively touch, caress, and kiss their baby's feet. Maybe that's because we instinctively know the soles of our baby's feet respond to our loving touch and help us connect deeply with them.

Not all nerve endings transmit the same information. For example, some sense light touch, others deep pressure, another set conveys temperature information, and others sense pain. Each of these is vital sensory information your baby needs to move and stay safe. Without those critical tactile senses, your baby will have trouble learning to move and walk.

We rarely think about what our feet tell us unless they become uncomfortable. We usually become aware of them when our toes are pinched or when we step on a sharp object. But even when we're unaware, we depend on those nerves in the soles of our feet to keep us mobile and safe.

Massaging your baby's feet can improve their blood circulation and even their digestion. In addition, you can tickle and excite your baby through the soles of their feet and kiss those pinky toes to convey love and comfort. So, take care of your baby's feet.

Ways to Encourage Your Baby's Development:

- Gently massage the soles of your baby's feet after bath time or diaper changes.
- While facing your baby, play peekaboo and cover your eyes with their feet.

Things to Remember:

You love it when I play "This Little Piggie" with your toes.
Your feet seem very sensitive/insensitive to touch.

Chapter 13

Grief

No one ever told me that grief felt so like fear.[1]

Tears of joy or tears of sadness? Sometimes when you're in those early days of motherhood, tears flow and you don't know why. But looking back, I realize I was dealing with grief, and that is still tough—even years later—to acknowledge. I had a beautiful adopted boy whom I adored. So, why would I be dealing with grief?

The answer to that question lies in the above quote by C. S. Lewis. When I first read the passage, it rang true. I was experiencing fear. First, I feared being unprepared to take care of a child. I was terrified of doing something wrong and harming my child forever. Second, I had stopped working full-time, and even though I had picked up part-time jobs I feared losing my career or my identity. These fears are embarrassing to admit—but they're true.

Before becoming a mom, I had spent all my adult years educating and training to become a physical therapist; that was my identity. Being a mother was something I also wanted, but I quickly realized that stay-at-home mothers aren't revered by American society. Sadly, those judgments often come from other women. Our culture minimizes the value of motherhood as a full-time role. Instead, women often are encouraged to elevate their career and to place their value to society on professional achievement.

Eventually, I realized I was grieving the loss of that cultural acceptance and value. Mothering doesn't come with pats on the back, promotions, or annual performance reviews with pay upgrades. Nor does it come with participation trophies.

So yes, I grieved without realizing what I was sad about until much later. Are you there? Motherhood is a lifelong job, and it's impossible to place a monetary value on it. While our culture may devalue full-time motherhood, it is the most important job in the world. Careers are rewarding, but they'll only fill a season or two in your adult life. Motherhood is a role for every season. Enjoy it. Go ahead and grieve the loss of who you were or thought you would be, but celebrate your new, essential role. Wear the mantle of motherhood confidently and proudly, regardless of what others say.

Ways to Encourage Your Baby's Development:

- Revisit and share your favorite nursery rhymes and books with your baby.
- Remind yourself that you can be fantastic at multiple things, but maybe not all at the same time. Make the most of this time with your baby.

Things to Remember:

My favorite childhood songs were

____.

Nursery rhymes with finger plays, such as "Itsy Bitsy Spider," teach the rhythms of language and how to imitate actions—vital skills for future academic success. So, sing those silly songs.

Chapter 14

Rockabye Baby

The words to the nursery rhyme first appeared in print in "Mother Goose's Melody." (London, c. 1765). The original author of the lyrics is in dispute.[1]

The nursery rhyme "Rockabye Baby" is widely known. While the original author of the lyrics and melody aren't clear, some of the words in the song are clearly not comforting to a baby. For example, "When the bough breaks, the cradle will fall / And down will come baby, cradle and all." Do young children pay attention to the words as much as adults do? I don't recall thinking about the meaning of the song's lyrics until I was much older. But I remember feeling loved and safe while Mama sang the song.

That's the point of singing simple songs to your baby. Nursery rhymes have uncomplicated, comforting melodies, and your voice singing them comforts your baby. Plus, the rocking motion that naturally accompanies the songs also calms and soothes.

You could make up your own words for the melody, and the result would be the same for your child—relaxation and sleep. And getting your baby to sleep is the whole point of the lullaby.

Of note, music can be either calming or stimulating. We know this without scientific proof. When we need to exercise, we select something upbeat. When we need sleep, we want slower, softer sounds. The rhythms and pace you choose for your baby are similar. Don't pick an up-tempo song if you want your baby to quieten down. So, sing the old lullabies or create new ones, if you like. The point is to enjoy the time together. Your baby will remember the comfort of your presence and your voice. They won't get hung up on the fact that some of the lyrics aren't child friendly.

Ways to Encourage Your Baby's Development:

- Play soft music with gentle rhythms when you want your baby to be calm or to sleep.
- Sing to your baby. The quality of your voice is unimportant. Sing now while they think everything about you is lovely.

Things to Remember:

Your favorite style of music is

____.

To get you to stop crying, I often turn on

____.

Chapter 15

Running on Empty

Running on empty, running on, running blind, running on, running into the sun but I'm running behind.[1]

Jackson Browne's old hit, "Running on Empty," sums up the feeling you probably have with your new baby. No sleep, eating on the run, rushing from one task to another in a mindless loop of time that never ends. Before long, you'll be singing that song's chorus and understanding it in an entirely new way.

Thankfully, most mothers have the innate ability to multitask, anticipate needs, and accomplish an amazing amount on little sleep and nourishment. But if you maintain this pace, you'll eventually hit a wall. I know this firsthand.

For many moms, exhaustion becomes the new normal. Busy reaches another level. Anxiety, an overwhelming sense of the need to control every detail of life—and for some, panic attacks and depression—may settle in when your physical and emotional tanks flash Empty.

For me, this exhaustion didn't hit for many years. But when it did, running on empty became a big problem—requiring an extended period of sleep and time to reprioritize life. To this day, achieving balance is a work in progress for me. You can't run on empty for long;

eventually you'll find yourself out of gas on the side of life's highway. So, take care of yourself because no one else can do it for you.

Ways to Encourage Your Baby's Development:

- Encourage your baby to look for you by calling for them at different times from various locations in the room.
- Carry your baby (aka baby wearing) frequently. Babies who spend a lot of time on their backs in carriers or other equipment are at higher risk of developing flat spots on the back of their heads. Babies whose mothers carry them are not.

Things to Remember:

I love watching you.
I'm amazed at how much ____________________ you produce.

Chapter 16

Lift Your Eyes

Lift your eyes and look to the heavens: Who created all these? He who brings out the starry host one by one, and calls them each by name. Because of his great power and mighty strength, not one of them is missing.[1]

Your baby can begin to do a minute or two of time on their tummy when they come home from the hospital, unless their doctor has instructed otherwise. Tummy time is essential for your baby to strengthen the muscles that will help them sit and walk one day. One of the first things your little one will learn while lying on their tummy is to lift their head and eyes to look around. Mastering this ability can take months of regular practice.

Lifting the head and eyes is one of the first and most important motor skills your baby learns. Even adults, if they're afraid or need help, revert to that earliest action and lift their eyes toward the heavens seeking assistance. We may look down and around first, seeing our mistakes and difficulties, but when we're out of answers, we lift our eyes, crying to God for assistance. We become like babies.

Your little one begins their journey in life by learning to look up to find you—their source of support and sustenance. During tummy-time play, provide various textures and sounds for your baby to look at and touch. Never leave your baby unattended and keep your eyes on them at all times. Be the reason your baby lifts their eyes to look around. You're their favorite toy during these early days of development.

Don't fret about keeping up with all your other tasks. These early months of your child's life fly by. One day soon, your baby will prefer another toy over you.

Did you know that the act of looking down tends to bring our emotions and spirits down? Think about that when you look down as you scroll through information on your phone. Looking down deflates our moods. Instead, lift your eyes and look around at the sunlit clouds or starry skies. You'll feel better.

Ways to Encourage Your Baby's Development:

- Work toward zero screen time for your baby. Screens include television and tablets, even if the show is educational. Watching screens is harmful to the development of your baby's eyesight.
- Take daily walks outside with your baby. Looking up at the sky or searching for honeysuckle is healthy for both of you. Nature is healing.

Things to Remember:

My baby ____________________tummy time.
Every day I'll walk outside (weather permitting) with my baby and talk about what we see, hear, and smell.

Chapter 17

Lay Down

I just want to lay down on a beach, let the sun hit my face and forget about absolutely everything.[1]

Mothering is exhausting. Yes, it's exhilarating and fun too, but let's be honest. Sometimes all you want to do is walk out the door and head somewhere, *anywhere*, where you can be alone without responsibilities.

Funny thing is, most moms report they miss their children when they do get away, even for a date night. That longing for your baby is normal, but it doesn't mean the brief getaway was unnecessary.

Babies never run out of needs. Screams of hunger or dirty diapers, and fussing to change positions, be held, or be rocked create an endless to-do list. And you'll soon notice that nothing on the list is for you: no nap time, no me time, no time to lie down and do nothing.

You may also notice that no one is helping unless you specifically ask. You may feel selfish for asking or angry that no one saw what you needed and took care of it.

Today, make a list of a few things you require. A few minutes in the bathroom alone or a girl's trip to the beach for some sunny relaxation. Fill your emotional tank because you won't be helpful to your baby when it runs empty. Schedule time to ponder what you can lay down, starting today.

Ways to Encourage Your Baby's Development:

- Lie down for a few minutes when your baby naps. Even if you don't sleep, take deep breaths and list reasons to be thankful.
- Lay down some activities—either stop doing them for a season or delegate them to someone who can assist. Scrolling through social media content consumes time but often doesn't make you feel better. Consider another activity, maybe one that engages your creative side.

Things to Remember:

The first time you smiled was on
______________________________. For most babies, this occurs around two months.
I'll lay down the following activities for a while:
____.

Chapter 18

Just a Whisper

Beginning at four to five months, many new sounds arise. We begin to hear fully resonant vowel sounds, and babies explore pitch and intensity in squealing, yelling, growling, whispering and raspberries.[1]

When your baby learns to whisper, it is so cute. You often don't understand what they say in their breathy little voice. Still, the intimacy of communication warms the heart. You and your snuggle bunny now share secrets.

Babbling sounds (oohs and aahs) begin in the first few months of life. Intentional whispering usually doesn't occur until around four to five months, but your baby will enjoy you imitating whatever sounds they make. For example, when your baby coos, coo back. If they say dadada, get at their eye level and say dadada to them. Repeating the sounds your little one makes shows them that communication is a back-and-forth activity. It requires eye contact and social engagement. Too many of today's babies lack these skills, but they're essential to future success. A home where everybody is doing their own screen thing creates an environment in which interactive communication and together time are infrequent or absent. As your baby learns to engage and talk, foster an environment that encourages more of it.

Ways to Encourage Your Baby's Development:

- Babble back and forth with your child. Act interested in what they say and pretend you understand what they're saying. Follow up with, "Oh really? Tell me more."
- Look at and speak with your baby frequently. Put down your phone or another electronic device as much as possible.

Things to Remember:

Your first sounds were

____.

Check your baby's hearing. Make sure your baby can hear. Many communication delays occur when hearing is impaired.

Chapter 19

I Hear You

Hearing is the "process, function, or power of perceiving sound; specifically: the special sense by which noises and tones are received as stimuli." Listening, on the other hand, means "to pay attention to sound; to hear something with thoughtful attention; and to give consideration."[1]

Have you ever felt like no one is listening to you? Maybe you feel ignored or you think no one cares. You talk, and the other person seems distracted or is looking down, scrolling their social media feed while you're emptying your heart.

Women often joke about men having selective hearing, and some boy moms also say, "He hears what he wants to hear." As a mother of two sons, I agree that selective hearing exists. But as a pediatric physical therapist who has worked with thousands of young girls, I can confidently say girls often only hear what they want to hear too.

Hearing and listening are two different concepts, but the phrase "I hear you" means "I am listening, and I care." Humans crave that attention and heartfelt hearing, especially when we feel unnoticed and sad.

Your baby may hear you call their name but may not act like they heard you. If this is a regular event, have a conversation with their doctor. Please don't assume they don't want to listen to you because they're too young for that. Babies are naturally in the phase of "it's all about me and my needs." Later, they should notice your needs.

In the meantime, journal your thoughts and concerns, pray, and talk with trusted girlfriends so you feel listened to and loved. As a new mom, you may feel used and emotionally drained, which often leads to feeling unloved. I hear you. I've felt that way too. You need someone to hear what you're dealing with—not fix it, just hear it.

Ways to Encourage Your Baby's Development:

- A quick way to check if your baby can hear is to get behind them where they cannot see you. On their right side, shake your keys or clap your hands. Do they turn to find the sound? Do the same thing to the left side. If they don't turn or respond to those sounds, talk to their doctor.
- Your baby also wants to be listened to, so put away distractions and make eye contact. Let them know you're listening, not just hearing them as you do something else.

Things to Remember:

I had your hearing checked on

____.

I'll schedule some time to either talk with my friends or journal about my feelings.

Chapter 20

Going Without Sleep

Sleep is like the unicorn—it is rumored to exist,
but I doubt I will see any.[1]

Going without sleep was my most challenging adjustment in the early days of motherhood. I need rest and lots of it. While I managed to keep up with all my responsibilities, I felt as if I was slogging through knee-deep mud most days.

Are you able to rest when you can? According to Amy Wolfson, PhD, in *The Women's Book of Sleep*, "The light from the computer or television can be very stimulating and keep you up."[2] This is also true for the light from your phone, so scrolling through social media at 3:00 a.m. is probably not helping you relax as much as you believe. Sometimes we don't realize how tense we are until the tension subsides. When I finally relaxed, I sensed how tense my body had felt all the previous years. Feeling rested was wonderful!

Your overall mental and physical health will improve with more rest. You may know that already, but you wonder how to get more sleep with all the baby needs tugging at you. Take a few deep breaths and lift your eyes from your phone. Stare out into space and allow yourself to picture a lake. Is the water choppy and churning? If so, can you make the lake surface calm enough to see your reflection?

Mental visualization exercises, like the one described above, can help you rest your mind even when you're awake. Practice these exercises, and you'll get better at quieting your thoughts.

Your baby needs you to be your best. So, make some changes this week. Your brain needs the reset that rest provides.

Ways to Encourage Your Baby's Development:

- Babies also need quiet mental time. Try turning off the television or background music during the day and allow total quiet to become comfortable for both of you.
- Busyness isn't a sign you're better at mothering. Instead, learn to delegate or eliminate unnecessary activities that steal time from resting your brain and body.

Things to Remember:

I love the cute baby sounds you make when you're happy.
Today, we turned off electronics for ________________________ of time. The quiet was ____________________________.

Chapter 21

Fussy

Some babies just have a whole lot more needs, and they express them much more passionately than others.[1]

Is there anything more alerting than a baby crying? The tone and pitch are impossible to ignore, even if the cries aren't coming from your baby. We've all sat on an airplane or in a waiting room when a baby cried. The entire episode was exhausting, especially for the parents.

Many times, babies fuss because they're uncomfortable. Usually, the problem is easily remedied—a dirty diaper, gas, hunger, or teething pain. Other times, the baby fusses to fuss, or so it seems.

Yes, they want attention, but they aren't doing it to get under your skin. They aren't being mean or spiteful; they're too young to have those intentions. They are unhappy.

Have you ever felt unhappy but didn't know why? You weren't hungry or sleepy. You could entertain yourself with plenty of activities available, but none of those seemed the right route to happiness. So, you fussed—griping and moaning about this or that. Maybe you felt sorry for yourself or maybe you were angry about what another person had or hadn't done.

Fussy

While a fussy baby will exhaust and frustrate you, offer grace and understanding anyway. Others are likely offering grace and patience to you and your occasional sharp tone or impatience. Again, babies are not intentionally trying to irritate you. Babies aren't capable of intentionally getting under your skin. They often need loving touch and attention. Maybe you crave that too?

Ways to Encourage Your Baby's Development:

- Give your baby a variety of teething rings to mouth and chew. Different feels and textures give your little one more sensations to explore and learn.
- Talk to your baby as you run errands or work around the house.

Things to Remember:

Your favorite toy is

____.

I often fuss about

____.

Chapter 22

Fisted Hands

Newborns clench their fists due to the palmar grasp reflex. This reflex is activated when something, like your finger, is placed into the baby's palm. The reflex typically goes away by five months of age.[1]

Most moms and dads instinctively explore their newborn baby's hands. First, you count their fingers and toes, then you place your finger in that tiny hand, and your baby's reflexive grasp releases a surge of connection and love. These emotions are natural. While science has never fully answered why babies have this reflex, it may be nature's way of bonding you to your baby. When that little hand grabs yours, it changes you. From that moment, you'll do whatever necessary to keep your child alive and well.

When adults encounter hard times—those moments when we're knocked to our knees with fear or fright—we automatically seek something to grab. In our panic, we seem to go back to the baby stage of grasping something we believe will save us. Our brains seem to know we need a higher power.

Be gentle if your baby's hands are difficult to open when you clean them. Talk with your child's doctor if your baby keeps their hands fisted most of the time and you cannot get them open for cleaning.

Fisted Hands

This fisted condition often occurs with premature babies or ones who had a difficult birth. It's also common if your baby is colicky or unable to calm down. If unsure, trust your mother's instinct and discuss with their doctor.

Ways to Encourage Your Baby's Development:

- Gently open your baby's hands and massage their palms. After a bath is the best time.
- Kiss their hands and palms.

Things to Remember:

The first thing I noticed about your hands was

____.

Your hands remind me of your __________________________hands.

Chapter 23

First Smile

Your baby will have a 'social' smile by 2 months. That is a smile made with the purpose to engage others. Smiles before this age are often reflexive or random.[1]

Those first baby smiles are precious, especially when your baby intentionally smiles at you. With the increased awareness of autism, this social skill is now tracked closely by pediatricians and mothers who, in years past, paid less attention to smiling and eye contact.

We are social creatures by nature. Even those of us who are introverts or prefer-to-be-alone types enjoy time with others. Not that we dislike other people or don't know they're there. On the contrary, many of us become anxious in social settings and seek comfort in solitude.

Talk with your child's doctor if your baby isn't smiling or making eye contact in a direct, purposeful fashion. Babies may have hearing deficits or social anxiety that contribute to social disengagement. Other times, they become focused on electronic screens and ignore people. Experts can assess if your baby has developmental delays. While it's frightening to face the possibility that your baby may have a problem, rest assured there are effective strategies that help. The earlier the intervention begins, the better the strategies work.

In the meantime, continue to engage with your baby face-to-face. Smiling, cooing, kissing, and frequently talking during the day are essential to your child's development. All of us like to engage with electronic entertainment, but that isn't healthy for young children. Children learn to communicate and socialize only by interacting directly with others. Unfortunately, delays in social and language skills occur in children who spend too much time on electronic screens, even when the game or TV show is educational.

Ways to Encourage Your Baby's Development:

- Work toward zero screen time in your home. Screens include televisions on in the background. Your child may not be able to hear you over the noise in the room.
- Offer your baby a child-safe mirror to encourage them to look at, touch, and kiss their image.

Things to Remember:

You first smiled intentionally at me on

____.

When you look in a mirror, you

____.

Chapter 24

Feeding Troubles

The American Academy of Pediatricians recommends babies drink breast milk exclusively for the first six months of life.[1]

Doctors recommend breastmilk as the best thing for your baby from birth to six months of age. The science clearly shows breastmilk provides the necessary nutrition and immunity your baby needs. Other benefits include comfort and skin-to-skin contact. As discussed in an earlier chapter, many mothers breastfeed easily, while others struggle. When you or your baby cannot sustain breastfeeding and must drink formula, you may feel profoundly dissatisfied and inadequate. Or you may feel free. How a mother feels about this topic varies wildly.

Many babies cannot get enough milk from the breast, which isn't always due to the mother not having enough milk. While some women produce excessive amounts of milk, others don't have enough. And breast size has nothing to do with milk volume.

Babies have trouble feeding in those critical early months for many reasons. For example, they can struggle with latching or become tired from sucking.

Feeding troubles are nothing new. From the beginning of time, mothers who didn't produce enough milk needed a wet nurse to feed their babies. Today, we have formulas and various nipples that make bottle feeding work for babies who need them.

If you or your baby has feeding troubles, you aren't abnormal, and neither is your baby. Don't receive and believe judgmental or unhelpful talk from others. The only thing that matters is your baby's health. Talk to your pediatrician or a lactation consultant. Get help.

WAYS TO ENCOURAGE YOUR BABY'S DEVELOPMENT:

- If your baby has digestive issues, talk to your baby's doctor. Your child may even have allergic reactions to a food you ate that was present in your breast milk.
- Talk to your pediatrician if your baby can only feed from one side. Your baby may have a lip tie or torticollis. Both these conditions can affect sucking and swallowing. They are treatable, and treatments work best if they're initiated early.

THINGS TO REMEMBER:

I love to listen to ____
while you are feeding.
I'm feeling ____________________________________ about how
breastfeeding is going.

Chapter 25

Eyes on Me

Let us fix our eyes on Jesus, the author and perfecter of our faith, who for the joy set before him endured the cross, scorning its shame, and sat down at the right hand of the throne of God.[1]

One of the first things your baby learns to identify is your face. This occurs within days or weeks after birth. Soon your baby will watch you move around the room. So, visual tracking is an important skill your child needs to see and explore the world. But as your little one masters looking around to find faces, did you know it's more complicated for your baby to fix their eyes, in a sustained way, to view something? Yes, it's easier to glance from one shiny object to another, if you will, than to focus intently on one item.

Knowing this about our eyes and the skill required to stay focused on one object makes the command for us to fix our eyes on Jesus even more enlightening. The word *fix* conveys a steady, steadfast watching. Have you thought about what your eyes are fixed on? What you look at most of the time says a lot about where you go and whom you follow. On what are your sights set?

Your baby will fix their eyes on you and trust your provision and guidance. Ask yourself, "What am I focused on, and where am I leading my child?" During my early days of motherhood, my eyes often focused on imaginary problems and fears of what could go wrong. As a result, my child may have sensed my unsteadiness.

Give your baby plenty of opportunities to fix their eyes on your face and soak up every moment. You want your child to learn that you are their safe place and first love. They can trust you. And give yourself time to discover what you most focus on and follow. Where you go is where you will lead your child.

Ways to Encourage Your Baby's Development:

- Peekaboo teaches your baby that you will return after briefly disappearing.
- Daily journaling and writing down all your worries can reveal how many things can distract you from being present in the moment. Being present and calm helps your baby's emotional development.

Things to Remember:

My biggest fear right now is

____.

I love watching you watch me.

Chapter 26

Different Cries

Crying is how babies express themselves. Newborn babies cry an average of two hours every day. From a few weeks old to around six weeks of age, the amount increases to three hours.[1]

I love every sound a baby makes except crying. Cooing sounds are lovely—even throaty gurgles. But not crying. A baby's cry is unnerving. For the crying to cease, someone must address the baby's needs. Ask any mother of a colicky baby or anyone who's been around a screaming baby. The cries of a baby are exasperating.

Babies begin with one cry which means, in essence, "Figure out what I need and help me." Eventually, your little one develops different cries to indicate various needs, such as a hungry cry versus a dirty-diaper cry. Mothers quickly pick up on what these diverse sounds mean.

While we instinctually know each cry is different, we learn the meanings through trial and error. We sense our baby needs something, and we figure it out. And in those moments when we've checked the diaper, fed and burped, and done everything else we can think of, we resort to holding and rocking.

When my babies were young, there is no telling how many hours I walked the floor thinking, *Everybody in the whole world is asleep right now, and I'm not.* Those days seemed like they would never end, but they did. And these days, filled with keeping your baby happy and quiet while you rock, feed, and change a million diapers, will also end. Your baby is just doing what babies do. They make sure their needs are met. Your baby isn't crying for any other reason.

Ways to Encourage Your Baby's Development:

- Keep a regular routine of diaper changes, feedings, and sleeping. Your baby will fuss less when they trust their needs will be met.
- Maintain a calm demeanor and voice level. Your baby may match your mood, so being upset won't help your baby calm down.

Things to Remember:

You were ________________ old when I realized you made different sounds to indicate various needs.

I need to sleep about ___________ hours a night to feel rested.

Chapter 27

Crossed Eyes

It is normal for your baby's eyes to sometimes cross. This usually goes away by 4–6 months of age.[1]

Newborns commonly have one or both eyes that cross. You may notice one of their eyes seems to go wonky when they gaze at your face. Why? In these early months, babies are learning how to control both eyes. Six muscles control each eye, so coordinating both eyes requires mastering the movements of twelve muscles. Your baby's eye muscles are gaining strength and coordination, which takes time.

Most babies will stop crossing their eyes by four to six months. So, if your baby still has issues after six months, discuss with their doctor. Early detection and intervention will ensure your baby's eyes work well.

You may have crossed your eyes as a game when you were young. Maybe someone told you to stop doing that or your eyes would get stuck. That fear was enough for me to stop doing it, even though the warning wasn't true.

But you know from having crossed your eyes that you can't see well and the world is unclear. For your newborn, that is how the world appears. Many babies have vision issues, and poor vision will impact your baby's development. Clear vision is vital.

While no one wants their baby to need eye surgery or glasses, the alternative is more undesirable. If you have any questions or concerns about how well your baby sees, seek an assessment from their doctor.

WAYS TO ENCOURAGE YOUR BABY'S DEVELOPMENT:

- Restrict fast-moving images from your baby's world. Focusing on electronic screens leads to eye strain and fatigue.
- If you use a baby mobile, place it where your baby looks directly overhead or slightly down toward their tummy to see it. Don't place it where your baby must crane their neck backward to see it.

THINGS TO REMEMBER:

Your eyes are the color of

____.

You passed your newborn vision screening on

__________________________.

Chapter 28

Born for a Purpose

For we are God's workmanship, created in Christ Jesus to do good works, for which God prepared in advance for us to do.[1]

Maybe you see no reason for life other than eating, drinking, working, and returning to the earth. I believe God intentionally created each of us for a divine purpose—no matter our imperfections. But being at peace with that fact took a long time.

I've treated thousands of children with various disabilities and have questioned God many times. Common inquiries included: Why do You allow babies to suffer? Why do accidents happen to children? What kind of God sits by and doesn't stop abuse? I'd love to tell you He gave me specific answers, but He didn't.

Still, I've come to rest in the hope that God is in control, and we aren't here to simply take up space until we die. Everything has a purpose. I believe when *your* mother held you, God already knew you'd be holding *your* baby one day. I see now that part of my ultimate purpose was to adopt my two beautiful sons. The journey through infertility and adoption wasn't my plan nor was an unexpected pregnancy their birth mothers' plan. But these situations were part of God's plan for my life and theirs.

While you certainly have other talents and ways to serve this world, motherhood will be your highest calling. But that's not the whole story. God also has a purpose for your baby's life, no matter the challenges ahead.

Trust me. Tomorrow will look a lot different than today. Continue to hope for the best and move forward.

Ways to Encourage Your Baby's Development:

- Visualize your baby as an adult. What kind of person do you want them to be?
- Write down a few priorities you can establish now that will impact the type of person you want them to become.

Things to Remember:

Do I believe that life, even one with disabilities, can be filled with purpose? Why?

____

____.

My baby has amazed me with how they've over-
come___________________________________.

Chapter 29

Being Held

Babies typically learn to self-soothe around 6 months.[1]

Eventually your baby can comfort themselves, and you won't have to pick them up and hold them each time they cry. But while cradling and comforting them may be something you love, you also need a break sometimes.

Maybe you work from home, are busy taking a shower, or wish your baby would find their thumb. While your little one should eventually learn to self-soothe, this important social skill is one we adapt as we age. We all seek ways to comfort ourselves.

Your baby will learn to cuddle a blanket or suck the pacifier while waiting for you to arrive. And in those harried moments as you juggle everybody's needs in the household, including your own, recall that life won't always be this way. One day, you'll drop your child off at preschool, and then as you return to the car, you may stuff your mouth with chocolates to soothe your fears.

Your child needs to learn to self-soothe, but did you know there's no scientific evidence proving that holding a baby a lot spoils them? During this season in life, go ahead and snuggle them. Enjoy the comfort it brings you both. One day, they won't want to remain in your arms, and you'll be left holding empty candy wrappers.

Ways to Encourage Your Baby's Development:

- To help your baby learn to self-soothe, comfort them in the crib without picking them up. Instead say something like, "Mommy's here. You're okay."
- Some babies don't sleep well because they aren't tired enough. Keep your baby physically active, playing on the floor or with you during their waking hours. Sitting and watching a screen won't burn off energy.

Things to Remember:

Your current favorite thing to do is

____.

Your sleep schedule is

____.

Chapter 30

Another Load

The average household washes 7.4 loads
—about 50 pounds of laundry—per week.[1]

Can we say a big thank-you for disposable diapers? Imagine how many loads of laundry you'd do without those disposable diapers? I don't even want to ponder the thought.

When my boys were younger, I was constantly climbing over mountains of laundry, and at times, my washing machine and dryer hummed nonstop. So many times the clean clothes never made it to the closet or chest of drawers. On some fast-paced days, we yanked those warm clothes directly out of the dryer and wiggled into them as we ran out the door.

When I think of how many times I took that washing machine and dryer for granted, I shake my head. In most parts of the world, mothers wash diapers and clothes by hand and hang them to dry. During a few of our worst hurricanes, my boys lived in their swim trunks for days because we had no electricity. When you have to wash clothes by hand, it's easy to talk yourself out of the need for constantly clean ones.

During your hectic days, as you bound over mountains of dirty sheets, spit-up bibs, and who-knows-what on your slacks, remind yourself to be thankful for a washing machine, either at home or at a nearby facility. How many loads per week do you do?

Ways to Encourage Your Baby's Development:

- Do your best to not get angry at your baby for being messy. It's simply a phase of their development.
- Expect your baby to be messy. They're learning about the world, and learning is always messy.

Things to Remember:

The most loads of laundry I have done in one day so far is

______________________________.

We use ________________________disposable diapers per day.

Chapter 31

A Little Extra

Down syndrome is a condition in which a person is born with an extra copy of chromosome 21.[1]

A little extra cream in the coffee or a touch more chocolate always seems like a good idea. But a tad more anxiety over your baby's development isn't so good, is it?

Most people know the cause of Down Syndrome is an extra set of chromosomes. They also understand that having an extra set of chromosome number twenty-one generates some differences in appearance and ability.

No one knows why God allows a child to have extra challenges. Finding peace about that has taken me years, but I have come to accept that He does allow struggles, even for babies. The Bible teaches He doesn't make mistakes, and I believe that. Therefore, if an extra set of challenges isn't an error, then He must have a plan. I have come to accept and trust His plan even when I don't understand it.

I wouldn't have designed life with these kinds of challenges, but I'm not the Creator. I'm a creation of the Creator, and my role is helping special-needs children and families. You and your baby also have roles to play. Maybe your role is to extend some extra understanding and acceptance for what you can't change. You baby's role may be to one day befriend a child with special needs, or if your little one has special challenges, they may teach others about courage. Over the many years of my career, losing hope seemed inevitable in some cases. But a double dose of patience and the courage to move forward with hope can enable you to expect blessings ahead. Simply take that extra step.

Ways to Encourage Your Baby's Development:

- Make a list of your baby's accomplishments and celebrate each one.
- Be your baby's advocate. No one else knows and loves this child as much as you.

Things to Remember:

I'll cultivate patience for

____.

Some things my baby does well are

____.

Chapter 32

Black and White

Black and white pictures or toys will keep your baby's interest longer than objects or pictures with lots of similar colors.[1]

At birth, your baby can see objects six to ten inches away but people or items further away will appear blurry. The activity your newborn loves and needs most during these early weeks and months is looking at faces and eyes. So, hold them often and give them tons of face time. In addition to faces and eyes, experts recommend using black-and-white cards or shapes in those early weeks. These high-contrast images hold your baby's attention longer.

While we love buying toys for our babies, your newborn doesn't require many items. Those stark black-and-white toys may seem ugly, and you may feel the urge for something prettier to show the depth of your devotion. While soft-colored walls and fabrics are fine, if you can't provide those at this time, rest easy knowing all your baby really needs is you.

Discard any guilt or thoughts such as *My nursery isn't as pretty as hers is.* Your baby cares only about your love and attention. Focus on what you do provide and build on that. Love will make up for most everything else.

Ways to Encourage Your Baby's Development:

- Place simple black-and-white cards within six to ten inches of your baby's face. Tell them what you see and point to eyes, noses, and other identifying characteristics.
- Provide a calm, safe, and loving environment. Make that your top priority.

Things to Remember:

I'm doing the best I can.
Your ________________is so cute.

Chapter 33

Something Is Wrong

At the end of the day, you know your children best. If you can rule out anxiety or fear as the foundation of a particular feeling or intuition, it's smart to trust that "mom gut" of yours.[1]

The number of times a mother has told me, "I knew something was wrong with my baby," has to total in the thousands at this point. Or the grandmother or foster mom says it. Either way, mothers tend to have accurate gut feelings. Some believe the mother's instinct occurs because of the bonding during pregnancy, which made the two individuals so connected that mom "just knows." However, my experience as an adoptive mother and accounts I've heard from other non-biological moms discount that common assumption. There is more to the connection than bonding during pregnancy.

Sometimes a mother senses something isn't quite right or her baby's behaviors seem off. Other times, mom, grandmom, or foster mom can't explain why they feel something is wrong. They just do. My children's pediatrician always assured me that if I suspected either of them to be sick to "go with my gut" and make an appointment. He'd decide if my child was ill. I respected that he validated my mother's instinct and didn't dismiss my concern as "in my head."

Something Is Wrong

I've helped thousands of babies and mothers. One affirmation I always give them is "trust your gut. If you suspect something is wrong, don't allow others to talk you out of it. Instead, get expert evaluations and advice. You may be worried over nothing, but then again, better to know than worry." Doctors and other medical professionals do their job, but they aren't always correct. You know your baby best, and if you sense something needs attention, persist until you get answers.

Ways to Encourage Your Baby's Development:

- Track your baby's milestones closely. Don't obsess over every little change but be informed.
- Remember that each child develops individually. Generally, however, most children meet major milestones around the same time. Therefore, if your child is behind, seek evaluations. Intervention works best when it begins early.

Things to Remember:

The doctor said you ____,
but I didn't agree.
Right now, I feel your development is

____.

Chapter 34

Born Too Early

Preterm birth is when a baby is born too early, before 37 weeks of pregnancy have been completed. In 2020, preterm birth affected 1 of every 10 infants born in the United States.[1]

For many years, I worked with premature babies in the neonatal intensive care unit at my local children's hospital. The youngest infant I treated was a twenty-five-week preemie. He was a record breaker for survival at that time. The complexity and beauty of a preterm baby always gave me a deep appreciation of the amazing fact that each of us begins from a single fertilized cell. The first fertilized cell quickly splits into two, then those two cells split into four, until a baby forms. During the baby's formation, some cells become skin, others bone, and each automatically becomes what it was meant to be. How this all occurs boggles my mind.

For most of us, myself included, seeing a preterm baby is jarring. Their fragility and vulnerability are evident—from their translucent skin to their small size. Many preemies struggle to maintain their essential vital functions, such as regulating their body temperature or breathing. When critical body functions aren't working as they should, we become acutely aware that life is fragile.

Born Too Early

If you gave birth to a preemie, adjust their age (from their due date) when checking if they're meeting their milestones. Until two years of age, the experts always determine your preemie's functional level based on their adjusted age.

Ways to Encourage Your Baby's Development:

- Remind yourself your premature baby is unique and may take longer to meet milestones than full-term babies.
- Many preemies require early intervention services to catch up with their same-aged peers. Get those services if your baby needs them. Your child deserves a strong start so they're ready for school.

Things to Remember:

Send thank-you notes to the doctors and nurses that helped your baby in the hospital.
My baby's journey inspires me
to____.

Chapter 35

Beware of Containers

Container Baby Syndrome may be identified when issues arise including delays achieving expected motor milestones such as rolling, sitting or standing; flat spots on the head due to lack of movement known as plagiocephaly; or tightness in the neck from keeping the head turned or tilted to one side known as torticollis.[1]

New mothers have many choices when shopping for their babies. The selection process can be overwhelming—from infant carriers, such as slings or packs; nursing pillows; floor or car seats; and infant swings. In order to complete other tasks, most moms want various safe places to put their babies. Since today's mother rarely has others available to hold the baby, she has no choice but to place the baby somewhere safe when she has other duties. The marketplace came to her rescue with tons of baby equipment. While these containers solve one problem, they also create new ones.

You may have never heard of Container Baby Syndrome, but it's an actual condition seen by many pediatric physical therapists. Delays in motor development often occur in babies who spend too much time safely supported in a container. Other conditions, such as flat spots on the head or a crooked neck, can also occur. Since newborns don't yet have good head control, lying in certain positions for long periods can lead to problems that may not be discovered until later. Limiting the use of containers helps your baby avoid these problems.

There are treatments for babies with Container Baby Syndrome; however, not every problem that develops is always completely resolved. The treatments are uncomfortable for your baby and costly for your budget. Therefore, prevention is best.

Ways to Encourage Your Baby's Development:

- Count how many hours a day your baby spends sleeping, playing, or resting while secured in equipment. Knowing the actual amount of time is eye-opening. Set a timer to remind you to change your baby's position.
- Offer more activities out of the containers to balance time in versus time out of them. Your baby needs many moments during the day when no pressure is placed on the back of their head. Laying your baby on their side to play is another option. But be safe and always keep your eyes on your baby.

Things to Remember:

My baby's favorite container to be in is

____.

Today, I'll begin rolling you on your side to play.

Chapter 36

Staying Warm

Babies can't adjust to temperature changes as well as adults. Babies can lose heat rapidly, nearly 4 times faster than an adult. Premature and low-birthweight babies don't have much body fat. Their bodies may not be ready to control their own temperature, even in a warm environment. Even full-term and healthy newborns may not be able to keep their body warm if the environment is too cold.[1]

Premature babies often have little to no body fat and struggle to stay warm. As a result, placing a cap on their heads helps them stay warmer. When a baby is cold, they burn calories to warm up. Preemies are already expending calories to breathe and eat. Ideally, a premature baby would still be in the womb, where these stresses wouldn't occur. But since the baby is outside the womb, they must work extra hard to survive. Without body fat to draw calories from, each calorie they eat is precious. So, if they require burning more calories to stay warm, the baby can't use those same calories to gain weight. Therefore, staying warm enough means more than being comfortable. Proper body temperature helps them gain weight and generate energy for other body functions.

Have you ever been cold? My family has enjoyed camping over the years, and we've spent many a cold night huddled in sleeping bags. We covered our heads with caps and our hands and feet with wool gloves and socks. Sometimes, we still shivered. If that situation had continued for a long time, we would've risked hypothermia. The possibility of hypothermia, a life-threatening condition, illustrates why staying warm enough is vital.

Ensure your baby stays warm—not hot, but not too cool. Since getting too cold is unsafe and can increase your baby's risk of Sudden Infant Death Syndrome (SIDS), make sure your home is warm enough for the baby. I've evaluated many low-weight babies in their homes. Many were cool to the touch and often irritable, and their moms wondered what was wrong. But after dressing the baby with another layer of clothing, most were warmer and calmer. We may forget how cool the air-conditioning and ceiling fans are to a baby with no body fat. Don't you tense your muscles and move more to warm up when you're cold? So, if you have a preemie, or even a baby who is underweight or on the light side, consider your baby's body temperature needs when you adjust your home's temperature.

WAYS TO ENCOURAGE YOUR BABY'S DEVELOPMENT:

- Maintain your baby's body temperature to help them gain weight and increase energy for growth.
- Don't let your baby sleep with anything on their head (unless instructed to do so by your doctor).

THINGS TO REMEMBER:

When you were born, your head was shaped like

_______________________________________.

When you're irritable, I'll remember to check if your body is too cool.

CHAPTER 37

PAT AND BAT

Your baby should be reaching for familiar objects by month 4, although some infants may begin reaching—for toys, for the dog, and of course, for their caregivers—by month 3.[1]

Most mothers use overhead mobiles to entertain their babies. For example, during baby's playtime on the floor, an overhead display of hanging toys offers enticing items to look at and grab. When your baby reaches out to pat or bat at items, they practice arm control and coordination. While the early movements are uncoordinated and involve more misses than hits, with time and practice, your baby should improve.

Another fun way to encourage your baby to look at and attempt to touch an overhead object is to tie a string around a lightweight toy. Slowly dangle the toy within your baby's reach and give them time to see and try to grab it. They may not attempt to reach for it until closer to two months of age, but watching the toy move slowly (and I emphasize slowly) in their line of sight is a beneficial play activity. Think of a cat trying to pat and bat a similar toy. The cat is learning to catch the object, and your baby is too.

When you play the pat-and-bat game or place the mobile overhead, ensure your baby doesn't have to crane their neck backward to see the toy. That extended position can strain your baby's eyes and neck. Instead, the ideal placement is above your baby's face or upper chest.

Ways to Encourage Your Baby's Development:

- Tie a string to a simple rubber teething ring, then slowly move the ring in front of your baby's face to encourage watching and reaching.
- Place one or both of your baby's hands on the breast or bottle during feedings. Doing this increases your baby's awareness of using their hands to feed themselves.

Things to Remember:

Your favorite things to pat or bat are

____.

You prefer watching ______________________________to looking at your overhead toys.

Chapter 38

Both Ends of the Bed

Flat head syndrome usually happens when a baby sleeps with the head turned to the same side during the first months of life. This causes a flat spot, either on one side or the back of the head.[1]

Some babies are born with a flat spot on their head, and others develop one later. While a flat area may appear for several reasons, a common cause is positional. While your baby was in the womb or after birth, they spent too much time with one part of their head pressed against something firm, like your pelvis. After birth, the crib mattress or carrier is pressed against the soft bone of your baby's skull, causing it to deform and flatten.

Most new moms are so busy and weary that they pay no attention to how their little one sleeps—whether they always lie on the same side of the head. After all, everyone has a preferred sleep position and may always go to sleep lying on the same side. But your baby's skull bones are still hardening, and spending long periods in certain positions can deform the bones. No parent wants that to occur. While some flattening of the skull can be corrected using a helmet, not all can. Do your best to prevent the problem from developing.

Ways to Encourage Your Baby's Development:

- Always lay your baby on their back to sleep. To encourage your child to look for you as you approach the crib, alternate which end of the crib you position them. Switching the position may decrease how long your baby lies in one place.
- Refrain from allowing your infant to sleep in a carrier or car seat. Flat on their back is the safest position.

Things to Remember:

You tend to sleep with your head turned

____.

I gently rub your head during the day, and you seem to

____.

Chapter 39

Feel the Rhythm

A sense of rhythm is defined as the ability to dance or play music or to stay with the beat of accompanying music.[1]

Most new moms have songs they love and want to introduce those rhythms to their babies. If you listened to music while pregnant, your baby picked up beats and bops in utero. Musical tastes vary wildly, so I won't speak ill of any style. Experts, however, recommend soft tones and gentle rhythms for babies because their senses are developing. Loud or rapid tones and rhythms can startle and overstimulate your baby, causing them to fuss and cry.

You want to move when you feel a certain rhythm. Why? Rhythms aren't only heard; they're also felt. The old-fashioned nursery rhymes have gentle melodies and predictable beats, which is why babies love them—a possible reason those songs have stood the test of time.

A fun way to play with your baby using nursery rhymes is to lay your baby on their back and gently cycle their legs like they're riding a bicycle. Keep up with the beat as you sing. Activities like this teach your baby how movements and rhythms blend. In addition, music and nursery rhymes will help your little one learn the language.

Ways to Encourage Your Baby's Development:

- Simple nursery rhymes are fun when you clap your baby's hands or gently pat their back to the beat.
- Introduce your baby to a variety of musical styles, including classical. See what they love.

Things to Remember:

You seem to enjoy ________________________music.
Some of my favorite songs are
____.

Chapter 40

Wait and See

Waiting is inevitable. Waiting with hope and courage is optional.[1]

Mothering requires a lot of waiting and seeing. As you travel through pregnancy or adoption, you often ask yourself, "Will my baby be okay?" Wait and see is the only answer. Later, when your baby has accidents or illnesses occur, again you'll ask, "Will my baby be okay?" No one enjoys living in wait-and-see mode.

I've treated hundreds of premature babies. During my job at the local children's hospital, I helped many preemies in the intensive care nursery. Every one of those babies and their families were living in wait-and-see mode. Some children were so young they couldn't drink from a bottle without respiratory or cardiac distress. Others were tense and had tight muscles, which may indicate a future diagnosis of cerebral palsy.

I've been in practice long enough to confidently say, "I've seen many such babies eventually accomplish things which astonished me." Those early days and months are too soon to make determinations about a child's future abilities. A multitude of changes can occur.

While I detest being told to wait and see as much as anyone else, when it comes to newborns, wait and see is sound advice. However, wait-and-see mode doesn't imply doing nothing. Seeking medical assessments, offering appropriate play activities, and learning as much as you can is my recommended action plan for a mom who's in a waiting period. Plus, while you wait, hang on to hope.

Ways to Encourage Your Baby's Development:

- Your baby needs encouragement. Never call your baby lazy. Lazy means unwilling to work. Being unwilling implies your baby can do the activity but prefers not to. In my experience, babies don't lie around doing nothing unless they can't move as they should. They're not unwilling; they're unable. Your baby may be doing their best.
- Recall how different you are today than when you were younger. If you can improve over time, so can your child. Hold on to hope.

Things to Remember:

The doctor recommended we wait and see about

____.

My favorite memories of your life so far are

____.

Section Two

Four To Six Months

Chapter 41

Looking at Hands

His little hands stole my heart
... and his little feet ran away with it.[1]

Every mother stares at, caresses, and kisses her baby's hands. She wonders what those little hands will do one day. Will they play the piano or build a car? Will they perform surgery or paint a masterpiece?

As your baby gets old enough to reach and grab, you stop dreaming about those hands performing neurosurgery or painting a masterpiece. Instead, you face the reality that all those hands are doing right now is making a mess you must clean up. Those chunky little hands soon tear, scatter, crush, drop, squeeze, and pinch. It is cute initially, and the family pet may love the floor droppings. But you tire of the mess quickly.

While you may not want to hear it, your baby will need years of practice to develop the coordination and skill to make less of a mess. Learning to pinch skin without hurting others, squeeze the juice box without squirting sticky liquid on the floor, and stack blocks instead of tossing them is how your baby learns. All this practice is trial and error.

Looking at Hands

Recall how often your hands have gotten you into trouble. Have you sent a mean text? Or hit back when you should have turned away? You may not have meant to harm, but you did.

During this stage of play, your baby learns how to control their hands. First, they master how to take items apart and dump them everywhere. Eventually, they figure out how to put something together and clean up—but not yet. Making a mess is a normal phase of learning. Everyone, even your baby, learns by trial and error. In the meantime, breathe deeply as you mop the kitchen floor for the millionth time, knowing this super messy phase will pass.

Ways to Encourage Your Baby's Development:

- Help your baby look at their hands. Say, "Your hands." Or use your child's name.
- Let your baby touch different textures (soft, hard, wet, dry, crinkly, etc.). Describe how those items feel. Don't allow your baby to handle hazardous materials.

Things to Remember:

Your hands are lovely.
You don't like touching

____.

Chapter 42

Mother's Voice

Just as your baby naturally prefers the human face over other visual patterns, they also prefer the human voice to other sounds. They will recognize and respond to those voices they hear most.[1]

Babies first hear and respond to your voice while in the womb. They know your voice and instinctively love when you talk to them. So, talking to your baby throughout the day—even about ordinary stuff like what you're cooking for dinner—is essential in your baby's development.

As they hear you chat, they learn the rhythm of language and how mom's voice sounds different than dad's deeper tone. They're building vocabulary even though it will be a while before they can say words. Children understand what is said to them long before they talk themselves. So talk.

I've evaluated a few young children who speak like cartoon characters because they spend too much time watching television or videos. I share this to illustrate that children copy what they hear most. It's much better if the voice they hear most is yours as you share how much you love them and celebrate their victories. The time for harsher tones and corrections comes later. For now, sing, talk, and enjoy each other's voices.

Ways to Encourage Your Baby's Development:

- When your baby coos, coo back. If they say ah, return with ah. They will talk more if they're listened to and encouraged.
- Baby talk is excellent, but so is talking to your child as you regularly speak. Do both.

Things to Remember:

Your first sound was

____.

You make cute faces when you talk.

Chapter 43

Oohs and Aahs

You know life has changed when going to the grocery store by yourself is a vacation.[1]

Most babies begin making ooh and aah sounds during the newborn phase. This language milestone is called cooing. You may automatically talk back to your baby with similar sounds. Most moms do. Often, what also occurs is you eventually realize you haven't had an adult conversation in a while. All your friends are at work or busy with their social calendars. Now that your baby may be sleeping more, you have time to realize you need some adult conversations.

You may desperately long to get away from the house. And you soon discover what all moms realize—the grocery store has become your refuge. There you can chit-chat with the clerk or others about something other than feedings and diaper changes. You realize you don't know what's happening in the world when you scan the magazine covers in the checkout line. Yes, you are in a new phase of life. But instead of moping, be thankful you are on this motherhood journey. This segment of your life is relatively short, although it feels like an eternity. Before long, you'll scratch your head, trying to recall at what age your baby began cooing and you gleefully cooed back. You'll laugh when you remember that going anywhere by yourself did, indeed, feel like a vacation.

Ways to Encourage Your Baby's Development:

- Take some time for yourself. Soak in a hot bath and say aah or ooh.
- Look in the mirror with your child. Coo back and forth with your baby, imitating their sounds. Be extra expressive, using your voice and face to show you're interested in what they're saying.

Things to Remember:

I'll get a baby-safe mirror we can enjoy together.
My favorite "me time" activity is

______________________________________.

Chapter 44

Peekaboo

Peekaboo is thought by developmental psychologists to demonstrate an infant's ability to understand object permanence. Object permanence is an important stage of cognitive development.[1]

The baby game of peekaboo is played around the world. Most new parents instinctively cover their faces with a blanket or hands, then quickly reveal themselves and exclaim, "Peekaboo! I see you!" Babies between four to six months usually love this game. Your baby may smile and giggle. When your child loves playing the game, you do more of it.

As with most games we play with babies, the silliness disguises the serious learning which occurs. For example, the game of peekaboo teaches your baby the important concept of object permanence—your baby learns that people and items still exist even when not seen or heard.

When your child is asleep in his room, you know they still exist even though you don't see them. But your baby is learning that you aren't permanently gone when they don't see or hear you. For your child to understand their pacifier isn't gone but may be under the blanket, they must grasp the concept of object permanence.

Another tidbit about peekaboo is that the back-and-forth play teaches your baby the rhythm and structure of social interactions. I see you, and you see me. I talk to you, and you respond. Back and forth is how we interact with each other, and peekaboo, while silly and fun, helps teach these critical cognitive skills.

Ways to Encourage Your Baby's Development:

- Play peekaboo with your baby. Encourage your baby to pull the blanket off your face.
- Cover your baby's rattle or bottle with a small towel or blanket and ask, "Where did it go?" Then encourage them to find the hidden item. When they do, say, "Here it is!"

Things to Remember:

I love playing peekaboo with you.
The first day I heard you laugh was

____.

Chapter 45

Who's That Baby?

Mirror play is also a way to nurture your child's developing self-awareness, which is a key part of their overall social-emotional development.[1]

Playing with babies between four and six months old is fun. Remember, these silly baby games teach important life concepts. For example, when your baby sees their image in the mirror, they don't know they're seeing a mirror image of their face. Instead, they think they see another baby. Babies don't recognize their image until around eighteen months. But these early games of looking in the mirror together help your child eventually identify their image and yours as well.

Sadly, I've evaluated many babies who have never looked into a mirror. Most homes have mirrors over the bathroom sink, and a few may have floor-length mirrors in the bedroom or hallway. These mirrors aren't easily accessible, nor are they shatter-resistant. My physical therapy treatment rooms always had a shatter-resistant mirror that began at the floor and went up at least four or five feet high. When babies first saw themselves, their expressions were priceless. Some who were fussing during tummy time looked up and stopped crying as they tried to figure out what they saw. Others reached out to touch or kiss the other baby. Mirrors are magical tools that help teach your baby their place in the world. One day when you ask your child, "Who's that baby?" they'll answer, "Me!"

Ways to Encourage Your Baby's Development:

- If possible, buy a shatter-resistant mirror to use with the baby. Point at their image and say, "Who's that baby?" Encourage your baby to point or pat their image.
- Make funny faces in the mirror to encourage your baby to watch your face closely. As your baby watches, they learn how to imitate facial expressions. Understanding facial expressions are an essential part of nonverbal communication.

Things to Remember:

We'll spend more time looking at each other in the mirror.
My baby will concentrate better if the television or smartphone remains out of sight.

Chapter 46

Where's Your Nose?

Knowing yourself is the beginning of all wisdom.[1]

Are you teaching your baby how to identify the parts of their body? One of the first and easiest ones to introduce is the nose. Since our noses are prominent features of our faces, babies tend to be interested in grabbing and touching them. Point to your child's nose and say, "Here's your nose," then point to your nose and say, "Here's my nose."

Dads enjoy this game and may make snorting noises to ramp up the fun. These activities hold your baby's attention and teach important concepts, such as naming and locating parts of their body.

Make sure your baby learns the names and locations of the parts of their bodies. One day they'll know what you mean when you ask, "Did you bump your head?" They won't understand your question if they don't know where their head is or what the word means.

Don't rely on electronic games or apps to teach your baby these concepts. Many mothers believe their child is learning during screen time, but technology is deceptive because children are retreating into self-directed entertainment and away from interpersonal interactions. The old-fashioned way remains superior.

Ways to Encourage Your Baby's Development:

- Adding funny sounds to touching noses increases the enjoyment.
- Bath time provides an opportunity to find belly buttons. When you wash your baby, tell your child what part of the body you're scrubbing. For example, "I'm washing your face."

Things to Remember:

When I ask you, "Where's your nose?" you touch your

____.

The first body part you learned to identify was

____.

Chapter 47

Learning to Calm Down

(24/7) once you sign on to be a mother,
that's the only shift they offer.[1]

Moms are universally sleep-deprived. Chronic fatigue often leads to short tempers and irritability. While all moms joke about how fatigue has caused bags under their eyes or their bodies to age ten years, no one has *real* answers on how to get more sleep. There are many opinions, but these vary wildly. Some say, "Put the baby in your bed," and others will scream, "Don't do that!" Others gleefully share that their baby goes back to sleep on their own and it was easy to teach, while their fellow mothers laugh and say, "Yeah, right."

No consensus exists on whether babies should be comforted or allowed to cry it out and calm themselves. With my son and my search for a good night's sleep, I eventually quit asking for advice because none of it was helpful.

Most babies can eventually perform some self-soothing behaviors, such as putting the pacifier back into their mouth. By six months, most can go eight hours without needing to eat, so you'd think they'd sleep all night. But they don't.

Learning to Calm Down

While it's essential to encourage your baby to self-soothe so you don't need to rush to assist every time, getting the right balance is a work in progress. We all need to learn how to calm ourselves, which is even harder when we're fatigued. So, take your sleep needs seriously and find what works for you and your baby. No matter what, always keep your baby safe.

Ways to Encourage Your Baby's Development:

- During the day, when your baby fusses, call out and reassure them you're there. Unless it's an emergency, slowly increase the time you wait to come to their aid.
- Experts recommend no electronic screens in your baby's room as blue light from the device can keep the baby awake.

Things to Remember:

I'll find what works for us and stop asking for advice.
Your favorite comfort item is

______________________________________.

Chapter 48

Kicking the Kitty

By 4–6 months, your baby now has more control of his head, hands and legs. He's able to roll over, push himself onto his arms and even kick at an object.[1]

Kicking begins as a reflexive movement. For example, touching the bottom of your baby's foot often causes your baby to kick. Typical motor development begins this way and advances to purposeful movement. For example, your newborn baby kicks randomly. By four to six months old, they intentionally kick to get a reaction, such as to activate a toy.

When your baby begins kicking the light-up toy at the foot of the crib, they're learning to play with toys. Cause-and-effect toys, such as those where you push a button and something happens, are appropriate for babies of this age. These toys also help your child learn where to place their foot or hand and how much force is required to make the toy work.

If you have pets, your baby may try to kick the kitty or dog. Be aware of the potential dangers of this activity. While your cat or dog may have been fine with your baby so far, when an unpredictable child begins to get into your pet's space, it may act aggressively. During my career, I've treated a few children who suffered grievous injuries when unexpectedly attacked by a family pet. Not one parent ever reported that they saw the aggressive reaction coming. Expect the unexpected with pets and keep your baby safe.

WAYS TO ENCOURAGE YOUR BABY'S DEVELOPMENT:

- Offer safe toys for your baby to kick, such as stuffed animals or mobiles.
- Encourage kicking, so your baby has strong legs.

THINGS TO REMEMBER:

Things you enjoy kicking are

____.

My baby should kick both legs equally well.

Chapter 49

Watching It Fall

Around 6 months old, babies start to delightfully drop objects—on purpose. This can be annoying for parents but it's actually important for tots to do.[1]

When you placed your finger in your baby's hand during those newborn days, they reflexively held on. In this development phase, they may not always grab your finger; they do it when they want to. Another skill they learn is to drop things on purpose. The only reason for this activity is to understand what happens. While this stage may be cute for a while, only the dog loves all the food dropped on the floor. But by watching objects fall, your baby creates their own cause-and-effect game. They drop the teething ring on the floor, and you pick it up. They think this game is fun.

They're not doing it to drive you batty; however, the game may exasperate you, especially if you're a clean freak like me. Tell yourself, "This is only a phase, this is only a phase, this is only a phase." Dropping items to watch them fall only lasts a short while.

Babies have to learn how things work, and it takes hours of practice to master certain skills, so offer patience and grace. After all, how long did it take you to learn how to hit a target or tie a bow? You made many mistakes, and your baby is no different. With time, they'll learn the skill and move on to something else.

Ways to Encourage Your Baby's Development:

- Drop a block into a bucket, then give your baby another block and say, "You do it," to encourage imitation. Laugh and giggle together.
- If your baby loves dropping food, place a plastic mat or shower curtain liner on the floor under the high chair so it's easier to clean up.

Things to Remember:

My baby loves to drop

____.

I'll buy wooden blocks for my baby, which will be a source of enjoyment for years.

Chapter 50

Baby Laughs

Many babies laugh out loud for the first time when they're 3 or 4 months old, although the first laugh may come later for many other babies.[1]

When your baby laughs out loud, you'll be delighted. Whether the result is a giggle or a belly laugh, you'll keep tickling that belly or sticking out your tongue to keep those lovely sounds coming. Laughing aloud is an important early indicator of social skills. Plus, it feels good.

We all know the adage "Laughter is the best medicine." When we laugh, our bodies release feel-good hormones in the bloodstream. Also, the physical act of laughing exercises and relaxes the diaphragm muscle. However, while vital for breathing, the diaphragm can also hold tension. You've felt it. Knots in the stomach or difficulty breathing are signs of anxiety affecting this muscle.

Laughter breaks up those knots, and the relaxation feels good. So, enjoy being silly with your baby and laugh together. It not only helps your baby's development of communication and social skills but also aids in emotional bonding and attachment.

If your baby isn't yet laughing, continue talking and engaging in many face-to-face interactions. Staring at your phone or other electronic devices communicates to your baby that you have better and more interesting things to do. Instead, engage with your little one and show them they're more important than any device or TV show.

Ways to Encourage Your Baby's Development:

- Continue encouraging your baby to look for you by calling their name from various locations in the room.
- Carry your baby frequently. As you laugh, they'll feel it. Snuggle, tickle, and kiss to show your baby how much you care. A loving touch can lead to lovely giggles.

Things to Remember:

You first laughed on

____.

What usually makes you giggle is

____.

Chapter 51

I Know You

By 3–4 months of age, a baby recognizes the parents and their vision keeps improving with each passing month.[1]

Babies are naturally attracted to faces more than anything else. Your baby wants to look at and know you. You'll see it in their eyes when they recognize you. Mom is their first love, and a deep, emotional connection forms when they see and remember who you are.

Sadly, this day of mutual connectedness may not have come for you. Some babies don't look directly at people, even their mom. When this occurs, it's worrisome. Fear of an autism diagnosis is on the minds of many mothers these days. And rightfully so, as the rate of autism has increased to a point where most people know someone affected. If your baby isn't making eye contact or looking at your face by four months old, please talk with your pediatrician.

Emotional attachment to your baby is tenuous when your baby doesn't demonstrate connection to you. If detachment is an issue, you may feel your baby needs you but doesn't care about you. While many moms may not admit this fear—even to themselves—it can lurk in their subconscious mind.

As a result of this repressed sadness, some mothers become angry or depressed. Others deny or push it into tomorrow's problems, hoping it will disappear. Unfortunately, repressed negative emotions can bubble up in the future. Your baby can't help how they act if they have a condition like autism. However, you can seek help, and receiving assistance earlier is best.

While what you most fear may never happen, your feelings *are* happening. Those emotions will impact how you care for and interact with your baby. In a private journal, write what is on your heart. Putting fears down on paper helps me realize what I'm hiding from myself. When I see what I'm hiding, I'm more likely to take positive steps and get help.

Ways to Encourage Your Baby's Development:

- Encourage eye-to-eye contact during conversations. Background noises from televisions or video games distract most babies and impair deeper person-to-person interactions.
- Many babies on the autism spectrum prefer to watch rapidly moving images, such as those on tablets, phones, or televisions. As a result, electronics can become an addiction that hinders the development of appropriate social skills.

Things to Remember:

I'll talk to your doctor about

____.

Today, I'll turn off the television when not actively watching a show.

Chapter 52

Time to Pivot

Babies typically begin pivoting in a circle on their belly around 6–7 months.[1]

When your baby learns to pivot in a circle on their belly, they've achieved an essential motor milestone. Two benefits of lots of tummy-time play for your baby are strengthening their back muscles and achieving early mobility. In addition, rolling over and pivoting to reach a favorite toy indicate your baby is gaining independence.

And independence is what mobility is all about. When your baby desires to look in the mirror, they can pivot to take a look. When the cat runs past, and your child wants to see where it went, they can turn around to check it out. They're beginning to explore and move around to see what they want to see.

Another meaning of the word *pivot* is to turn around on an opinion. Sometimes adults pivot on issues or decisions. Maybe you once believed one thing, and now you have redirected to another position. For instance, did you once say to yourself, "My child will never ..." and now find yourself thinking otherwise? Mothering is a humbling experience.

Time to Pivot

Learning to pivot is both good and bad for your baby, depending on how you view this milestone. For your baby, learning to pivot leads to greater mobility and increased access to danger. For example, they might spin around and find a battery on the floor. If they put it in their mouth and choke, that's bad. Enjoy your baby's newfound mobility, as it is an outstanding achievement. But prepare the play areas so they can explore safely. You can't be too careful. Get down on the floor at your baby's eye level and see what dangers are there. From that viewpoint, you can see how perilous your home can be.

Ways to Encourage Your Baby's Development:

- A firm, padded play mat allows your baby to move around safely. Avoid slippery or plush surfaces, as your baby can become entangled.
- Position your baby's teethers, rattles, and baby-safe books around the play area. Doing this will encourage your baby to pivot and figure out how to get to another toy.

Things to Remember:

You began pivoting on your belly on

____.

The most dangerous object I found when I checked your floor play area was ________________.

Chapter 53

Arms Up

Typically, by the end of 9 months, your baby may be able to lift arms to be picked up.[1]

One of the earliest ways your baby communicates with you is leaning and reaching for you. You know they want to be picked up when they reach for you. By around six months, most babies reach their arms when approached. It'll be a few more months before your child lifts their arms to be picked up. Regardless, this action warms your heart, and it may also make you aware that your baby is gaining some independence. Finally, they're physically moving to get what they want—you.

The act of reaching to be picked up is called a gesture. Gestures are early methods of communication. Most adults instinctively use and understand these gestures. For example, when your fussy baby reaches up, no one has to tell you what they want, right? You'll pick them up because you know they need comforting.

Gestures are important ways your baby communicates. Look for early ones, such as when they shake their head or give you a toy when you extend your hand. When you hold out your upturned hand, this gesture means "hand me what you're holding."

Arms Up

Adults use gestures without realizing it. For example, shaking your head no or reaching out when you want a hug are ways we communicate. As you say words to your baby, add the gesture, so they learn both gestures and words. For example, if they don't reach for you, while you reach for them say, "Reach." Don't expect them to comply or withhold what they want unless they gesture. Instead, begin to gesture and say the words during your daily routine. They'll eventually associate the gesture with the words.

Ways to Encourage Your Baby's Development:

- Say "arms up" or "reach" as you reach for your baby. When they see your gestures, they'll try to model those actions.
- Offer your upturned hand and see if your baby automatically reaches back. Your tot may hand you what they're holding. In addition, you can say, "Give it," to add more vocabulary to the dialogue.

Things to Remember:

You began reaching for me on

____.

My favorite outfit for you right now is

______________________________.

Chapter 54

Reaching and Grasping

Sometimes all it takes is a little hand reaching to hold yours, to remind you, without a doubt, that these are the best days of your life.[1]

When a baby extends their hand toward me, I automatically reach for their hand. Reaching out is an early motor pattern that allows your baby to touch and explore people and objects. Since our hands are so sensitive to understanding how items feel when we touch them, we use our hands to figure out the world. We make decisions about what we like to touch and what we dislike. Babies are the same.

Since the skin of a baby's hand is still soft and uncalloused, they're more sensitive to what they touch. For example, I can tolerate stroking my hand across the sand. However, babies often recoil from certain textures or other sensations. We chuckle at first, until this extreme reaction prevents them from reaching and touching during play. Having some aversion to touching certain objects is typical for babies. However, some children have severe reactions that warrant further discussion. Two early signs of sensory hypersensitivity are (1) your baby gags or vomits when certain items are touched, or (2) your child screams and recoils to escape what's unpleasant.

If you suspect your baby isn't reaching out or grasping objects because they seem overly sensitive, talk with their doctor. Some overreactions will work out over time, but others may need further assessment. Babies can learn to tolerate and even enjoy touching items they once detested.

Ways to Encourage Your Baby's Development:

- Offer your baby a variety of objects to reach for and touch, such as soft blankets, crinkly books, cool water, or pureed foods.
- Allow your baby to have messy hands during feedings to increase their tolerance for textures. Let them spread some of these foods on their face to teach them that these textures aren't harmful.

Things to Remember:

You seem to enjoy touching

____.

You don't enjoy touching

____.

Chapter 55

Praying Hands

By 3 months of age, infants can bring their hands together in front of their face.[1]

When your baby learns to bring their hands together, it often looks like they're praying. And it's so stinking cute!

A significant milestone has been achieved when your baby can get their hands together to hold an object or clap. Newborn babies exhibit movements that are primarily reflexive and unintentional. For example, when you put your finger in your baby's hand, they hold on. As mentioned earlier, as they get a little older, they won't automatically grab your finger. The ability to choose whether to grasp shows your baby controls their hand. Also, newborns have many movement patterns where one side of the body does one thing while the other half does another. For example, your baby may keep one arm straight and the other bent. These movements are asymmetrical and expected. However, by six months, many of those asymmetrical and reflexive motor patterns have progressed into symmetrical and intentional ones. Getting the hands together is a sign your baby is doing the same movement with each hand and doing the action on purpose.

In addition, when your tot gets their hands together, this indicates they can reach both hands to the midline of their body. Midline activities, such as clapping hands or holding a bottle, suggest that the right and left hemispheres of your child's brain are communicating. Our more sophisticated movements occur at the midline. Therefore, creating opportunities for both right- and left-brain hemispheres to work together more closely is desirable. Many baby games we know, such as clapping hands or playing patty-cake, meet this criteria.

Talk to your child's doctor if your baby isn't yet getting their hands together at the midline or if they keep them clasped together most of the time. They should be able to move them in all directions and get them together occasionally.

WAYS TO ENCOURAGE YOUR BABY'S DEVELOPMENT:

- Clap hands with your baby. Help them clap by holding your baby's hands together.
- Play patty-cake with your child. Don't expect them to do all the hand movements yet. Instead, help them do the motions and make it fun.

THINGS TO REMEMBER:

You first put your hands together on

____.

I'll talk to the doctor about

____.

Chapter 56

Shake, Rattle, and Roll

"Shake, Rattle, and Roll," a song written by Joe Turner in 1954, rocketed to legacy status when recorded by Bill Haley & the Comets later in 1954. In the 1990s, Elvis also had a hit with this song.[1]

Much of your baby's play in the first six months could be described as a lot of shake, rattle, and roll. Shaking, mouthing, and dropping rattles occupies hours of your baby's first play activities. For example, during playtime on the floor, your child learns to roll over, by accident at first, to change positions. Soon, they intentionally roll over to reach something they want to touch.

With this increased independence will come broken toys, hurt feelings, bumps, and bruises. Be alert to keep your baby safe from bumping into or banging against sharp edges. They'll also cry many tears over toys dropped out of reach.

Adults do the same things repeatedly, too. Have you ever banged up against the same unhealthy thoughts over and over? Or do you keep stubbing your toe on the bedframe even though you know it's there?

Hopefully, we eventually learn to steer clear of danger and stop trying to make things happen on our terms. Your baby is learning that when they let go of the teething ring, it falls out of reach. They'll do this same thing hundreds of times before they "get it." Be patient. This is just another example of everyday activities not going as planned.

Ways to Encourage Your Baby's Development:

- Listen to Elvis sing "Shake, Rattle, and Roll" and see how your baby reacts or play other music your child enjoys.
- By six months, most babies reach for toys or people.

Things to Remember:

Your favorite song or musical style is

____.

The hand you prefer to use when banging toys is the

____________________hand.

Chapter 57

Into the Mouth

Babies put everything into their mouths as a part of learning and development. It also helps their bodies get stronger and better able to keep them healthy.[1]

At first, it's cute when your baby mouths their fingers, rattles, and teething rings. But eventually, it becomes exhausting because you must remain vigilant to prevent them from mouthing electrical cords, dog biscuits, or sharp objects.

Babies mouth objects to taste and feel them. They also mouth and gnaw on toys when teething, and some children mouth things even when they're much older. For many such children, this continued mouthing is either a form of exploration or a way to calm themselves.

The mouth has an extremely high concentration of sensory nerve endings that provide a lot of information. Our mouths tell us how something tastes—whether it is sweet, salty, sour, or bitter—and whether it is pleasant or noxious. Specific nerves tell us how hot or cold the items are and whether there's a small or large volume in our mouths. How things smell is also tied to taste, so babies may be exploring smells while tasting everything. Later, your baby will learn the words we use to describe those memories. Words such as *bumpy, lumpy, sandy*, or *slimy* will eventually describe those sensory memories your child is making now.

Mouthing objects is typical; it's also vital to your baby's development. Keep your baby safe but also understand why these activities are essential to your baby's brain development. Mouthing isn't a mindless activity to a child.

Adults often mouth things, too, such as chewing on the top of a pen or sucking on a breath mint. While we often do it mindlessly to focus our thoughts or distract ourselves, sometimes we reach for food to feed an emotion. For example, we may push down unpleasant feelings by munching on salty crackers or slurping ice cream. Mouthing objects doesn't cease as we age—the reasons for it change. Keep your baby safe during this phase and think twice about using snacks to keep yourself entertained.

WAYS TO ENCOURAGE YOUR BABY'S DEVELOPMENT:

- Offer a variety of safe toys your baby can put in their mouth to chew. Try different textures. You can even put some of them in the refrigerator to add a cooler temperature to your baby's sensory diet.
- Offer thick cardboard or padded books for your baby. Your baby can explore, even chew, these books safely.

THINGS TO REMEMBER:

Your favorite toy to chew on is

____.

I'll ensure my baby can't reach any cords from electrical appliances or window coverings.

Chapter 58

Hand to Hand

Between five and seven months of age, most babies have mastered being able to transfer a toy or other object from one hand to the other.[1]

The hand is a complex part of the body comprised of over thirty muscles working with precision to accomplish tasks. Infants learn how to use their hands by first batting and roughly grabbing objects. Eventually, after months of practice, they know to pick up and hold a ring or something similar. Next, they may try to put it in their mouth or bang it against something. Finally, after a few more months of practice, your baby begins to transfer the toy from one hand to the other.

These accomplishments may seem of little consequence to most moms. But to a developmental expert like a physical therapist, these milestones are pivotal for your baby to move forward and improve by using both hands together.

Banging toys together or switching hands with a toy also means your baby's brain has reached a higher level of development. Both the right and left sides of their brain must communicate back and forth to accomplish these tasks.

Hand to Hand

If both hands can't work together in this back-and-forth manner, your baby will struggle to learn how to get dressed, drive a riding toy, or even hold down the paper while writing. Of course, experts may find ways to help a child if they don't master these skills, but preventing these struggles is much better.

Our hands are essential for us to do many things. Providing a variety of toys for your baby to pick up and change hands with is ideal. Avoid using electronic toys or ones that rely on batteries. Your child will lose interest in them when the lights don't work or the music doesn't play. Instead try blocks, balls, books, and containers of various sizes. These simple toys offer more ways for your baby to learn good hand coordination.

Ways to Encourage Your Baby's Development:

- Offer various sizes of blocks, balls, and containers. Your baby will enjoy putting items into the bucket or dumping them out.
- Place the toys in your baby's right hand sometimes and in the left at other times. Your baby is learning to use both hands at this age.

Things to Remember:

The day you began moving a toy from one hand to the other was on

________________.

Your favorite toy right now is

____.

Chapter 59

Babbling

Babbling is the use of repeated syllables over and over like 'bababa' with specific meaning. Later on, babbling turns into baby jargon or 'nonsense speech.'[1]

The word *babble* can also refer to chattering or mumbling about something of no importance, such as kids babbling in the background. The word also sounds like the word *Babel* from the Bible. In that account, God destroyed the Tower of Babel and caused all the people who once shared a language to speak different languages, thus creating disunity and an inability to understand one another. When you wonder what your baby is babbling about, you may feel you each speak a different language.

Babies babble as they learn to form and produce consonant-vowel combinations. These early bababas or dadadas later evolve into more complex sounds and words. Later, babbles progress to baby jargon, which experts call nonsensical speech because it sounds like a foreign language. You may not understand what your baby babbles about, but you will probably find it adorable. So, when your little one is babbling on about this and that, and you have no earthly idea what they're talking about, pretend you do.

Babbling

When they say dadada or bababa, say dadada or bababa back to them. Act interested. Maybe you could say, "Tell me more," and see if they continue talking. Babies love to be listened to; truth be told, we all do.

Ways to Encourage Your Baby's Development:

- When your baby says bababa, you should repeat bababa back. Speaking to your child using adult words is fine, but talking baby talk to your child encourages more talking. After all, you're speaking their language.
- Let your baby see themselves babbling while looking at their reflection in a mirror. They may watch your mouth as you say words, which is helpful as they learn to pronounce actual words.

Things to Remember:

Your first babble sounds are

____.

I wish you'd say the word

____.

Chapter 60

Rolling Over

By six months of age, most babies can roll over in both directions —tummy to back and back to tummy.[1]

The first few times your baby rolls over—usually from tummy to back—are accidental. Your little one has learned to lean from one side to the other; when they do, they flip over. Your child may act surprised or even cry those first few times since the rapid movement can startle them.

But soon they become accustomed to the sudden change in position and "go with the flow." It takes a bit longer to gain enough strength and control to roll from their back to their tummy because that movement can't happen accidentally.

Rolling in both directions is a huge achievement for your baby and sets them on a path toward even more mobility. While not all babies achieve this bidirectional rolling by six months, it shouldn't take much longer.

When they do learn to roll back and forth, you may return to the room and find your baby has rolled across the floor and gotten into trouble. Time for more safety measures. Certain areas, stairs especially, must be cordoned off so your child can't roll into danger.

Rolling Over

Rolling is an indicator your baby can rotate, and rotational movements are considered advanced. Celebrate that your child can perform the foundational actions they'll need to crawl, walk, and run one day.

Ways to Encourage Your Baby's Development:

- Give your baby lots of playtime on the floor. Ensure your baby has safe areas to roll around and not get hurt.
- Limit the use of baby walkers, stationary play stations, or jumpers. These types of equipment block the development of the rotational control needed for future crawling and walking.

Things to Remember:

You began rolling on

____.

I'll ensure that you can roll in both directions, right and left.

CHAPTER 61

SITTING UP

There are seasons in life. Don't ever let anyone try to deny you the joy of one season because they believe you should stay in another season. ... Listen to yourself. Trust your instincts. Keep your perspective.[1]

Since birth, your baby has been changing moment by moment. They're learning and growing each day as they reach and achieve new developmental milestones. So, while we may not view those phases as seasons, we could.

If your baby is learning how to sit up, they're in a new season of life. They now have an elevated perspective where they can see and grasp objects previously beyond reach. But unfortunately, they can also fall and get hurt, especially if their head hits something hard or sharp.

With each new milestone, your baby gains independence and takes on more risk. But life is about both of those. As adults, we love to do what we see fit without others controlling us. Sadly, some may use this independence to flee responsibilities. However, we prefer the freedom to do what we want.

As a new mother, you're also in a new season. In this one, you care for a baby with rapidly changing habits as well as increasing mobility and danger, and you have a kitchen floor that won't stay clean. From newborn days to now, life has been a roller coaster.

Take time to view life from your higher perspective as the mother of a child who may be midway to one year old. What have you learned about yourself? Have you enjoyed this time with your baby, or has it been more challenging than you prefer? My children's pediatrician once said God knew what He was doing when He allowed babies not to remember how hard the first year would be. If adults struggled that much, we'd never stop complaining about it. I think he was correct about that.

WAYS TO ENCOURAGE YOUR BABY'S DEVELOPMENT:

- Place pillows around your baby while they're sitting. If they fall, the extra padding can prevent injury.
- Sit on the floor with your baby and place them between your legs. They can practice their balance, and you can catch them if necessary.

THINGS TO REMEMBER:

You learned to sit by yourself on

____.

I'll sit on the floor with you at least once each day.

Chapter 62

Sucking on Toes

There are over 200,000 nerve endings in each foot. [1]

When your baby touches their chunky feet, they may pull them toward their mouth so they can suck on their toes. Sucking on toes and grabbing those feet may seem like child's play. Most parents think it's cute. And it is, but more is going on than you realize.

What seems like play is important work. For example, when your baby grabs their feet, they realize those are their feet. As they touch and mouth their toes, all those nerve endings in their feet, hands, and mouth are sending their brain tons of information.

All that knowledge lets your baby know those appendages are attached to their body. Making this tactile and visual connection to the lower half of their body will be essential as they learn to pull off socks or put on shoes.

The nursery rhyme, "This Little Piggy Went to Market," remains an effective way to teach your baby about each toe. And we all know the anticipation that builds as they wait for the silly ending. "And this little piggy cried 'wee, wee, wee' all the way home!" is fun for everyone.

Children love silliness and simple musical melodies. We remember those longer than more detailed information. So, tickle those toes and kiss those plump heels. Significant development is happening as your baby sucks on their toes.

Ways to Encourage Your Baby's Development:

- During bath time, play "This Little Piggy Went to Market" with your baby's feet.
- After diaper changes, help your baby grab their toes. If they struggle, hold their hands on their feet so they can touch them.

Things to Remember:

When we play "This Little Piggy Went to Market," you

____________________________.

I love kissing your toes.

Chapter 63

Splash Time

At around 5 months old, a baby's ability to see how far an object is from them (called depth perception) has developed more fully. They are seeing the world in 3 dimensions (3-D) more completely. They get better at reaching for objects both near and far. They also have good color vision at this point, though not quite as fully developed as an adult's.[1]

Your baby's visual development is rapidly coming along during these early months of life. They watch you walk across the room and enjoy seeing colors for the first time. Providing variety in your child's experiences is important.

One such way is to enjoy the water. As your baby sits in the tub, they can bat at floating toys and learn how they move and what it takes to touch them. They may like splashing their hands on a water-filled cookie sheet while sitting in a high chair. A yellow duckie or red ball bobbing and weaving can offer minutes of healthy play for your baby. But, of course, when you combine babies and water, safety is essential. A baby can drown in an inch or two of water, so stay nearby.

We take for granted our baby's visual development will properly occur when we allow our babies to watch videos on smartphones or tablets. But when babies play on electronic devices, they don't learn depth perception or how to see in three dimensions. For example, if your baby plays with a block, they learn to see in three dimensions. Objects on screens are two-dimensional.

So splash in water, touch and squeeze a real rubber duckie. Your baby's visual, brain, and motor development will benefit from these hands-on activities.

Ways to Encourage Your Baby's Development:

- Use everyday objects in the tub, such as measuring cups, spoons, or funnels. Splashing, pouring, dumping, and watching are all brain-building opportunities your baby will love, and so will your wallet.
- Place thinly sliced limes or lemons in a plastic storage bag. Fill the bag with water, so the slices float. Zip the bag shut and let your baby touch, pat, and squeeze. Double-bag so nothing leaks.

Things to Remember:

Your favorite bath-time toys are

____.

I'll add some water activities to your day.

Chapter 64

Bouncing

Any jumper, also known as a bouncer, should keep your baby's legs in a natural, relaxed position. Jumpers that keep the legs open can put pressure on their hips and can cause problems in hip development.[1]

Baby bouncers are popular with parents and babies. Over the years, hundreds of moms and grandmoms have shared with me, "They love their jumper!" But knowing what I do about baby development, I cringe. Just because the baby and caretakers love the bouncer doesn't mean the bouncer is a healthy choice.

When your child sits in a bouncer seat, the sling seat usually positions the legs wide apart. This position is unsuitable for your baby for extended periods. Ten or fifteen minutes twice a day should be safe, but leaving them in that position while you cook dinner or do a thirty-minute workout is too long.

Your baby's hip joint can be easily damaged at this young age because the socket isn't deeply seated. Adult hips are difficult to dislocate because the thigh bone is solidly seated inside the pelvis. Standing and walking cause the hip socket to form into a stable joint. Since your baby isn't yet walking or standing for long periods, the hip socket is still in the development phase. Therefore, putting those hips in non-ideal positions for extended periods can damage the joint.

Jumping and bouncing put pressure and strain on the muscles and ligaments of your baby's hip joints. These weak muscles and ligaments are still developing. Although many parents believe jumping and bouncing strengthen those legs, the equipment your baby uses to jump creates undue pressure on their hips. Jumping isn't normal for a baby of this age because they aren't walking yet. Walking and running develop before jumping on a typical developmental timeline. The ability to jump usually doesn't develop until your baby is around two years old. A safer alternative to jumpers or bouncers is lots of playtime on the floor.

Ways to Encourage Your Baby's Development:

- Bounce your baby on your lap and sing songs. Your baby's hips are safer when you control this activity rather than using the equipment.
- If you use a bouncer or jumper, don't exceed ten to fifteen minutes each session, and only do two bouncer sessions per day.

Things to Remember:

I'll get a playpen so you can be safe while you move around.
You don't like to put weight on your legs. I should talk to the doctor about this.

Chapter 65

Clap, Clap

Clapping usually happens around 9 months of age, but that's just an average.[1]

While your baby may not clap their hands during the four-to-six-months age range, they are beginning to get their hands together. As they gain the coordination to touch their hands together at the midline of their body, they're well on their way to clapping when they're happy.

You may have already started helping your child clap their hands. Most of us grab our tot's hands and clap them. Silly baby games, such as patty-cake, help make learning fun. And when it comes to how babies learn best, fun is essential.

Some babies learn these games earlier, others later. These ranges are typical. However, suppose your baby shows no signs of getting their hands together at the midline and resists your attempts to help. In that case, they may have some sensory defensiveness.

If they pull away when you hold their hands, try holding their arms at the elbows and help them clap. The skin around the elbows has fewer nerve endings than the hands, and your baby may prefer your assistance. Try this a few times but don't make it a battle. Always make it playful.

Babies who consistently resist getting their hands together to clap or touch the bottle may need further assessment to ensure development is on track. Most often, there are easy ways to help your baby. Still, a more detailed evaluation is needed to discover the exact approach.

WAYS TO ENCOURAGE YOUR BABY'S DEVELOPMENT:

- Babies learn by imitating the behaviors of others. For example, clap your hands when you are happy and act happy. Your baby learns what they see.
- Say, "Clap, clap!" as you help them clap. Continue saying the word that describes the movement. Babies need lots of repetition to learn the names of objects (nouns) and actions (verbs).

THINGS TO REMEMBER:

When we clap your hands together, you_________________________it. The song "When You're Happy and You Know It" teaches babies and toddlers clapping and other motor actions.

Chapter 66

Holding the Bottle

Your little one may be up to the task at around 6 months and possibly later up to 10 months, but don't be surprised if he doesn't fit neatly within the norm.[1]

Earlier in the book, I wrote that you'd want your baby to hold their own bottle one day. I also shared that your feelings surrounding the time spent feeding your child may move from "I love this so much!" to "When are they going to hold their bottle?"

Maybe you're not there yet, and not everyone feels that way. For many mothers, though, life gets going, and we must multitask to accomplish each day's to-do list. When your child can hold their bottle, you'll fill the time with other responsibilities.

Some babies reach for the bottle from the early days, and others never try to hold it. If your baby is one of the latter, bring their hands to the bottle and hold their hands there as they drink. Hand-over-hand assistance is one way to teach them. If their hands are fisted, gently open them and place the palms on the bottle. Then hold them that way as they feed.

Expect your baby to need some time to adjust to this new position. When their hands are on the bottle, the way they suck and swallow will change because those muscles are now aligned differently. These changes are helpful because your baby needs to strengthen their mouth and neck muscles to work well in all positions.

Ways to Encourage Your Baby's Development:

- Begin with smaller bottles, such as four-ounce or preemie bottles. Smaller bottles are easier for your baby to hold and lift because they weigh less.
- Never prop the bottle and leave your baby to feed unsupervised. Always have eyes on your baby.

Things to Remember:

I'll buy some small bottles to help you learn how to hold your bottle.
I'll talk to the doctor about how you're doing with holding your bottle.

Chapter 67

Call My Name

While your baby may recognize their name as early as 4 to 6 months, saying their name and the names of others may take until somewhere between 18 months and 24 months.[1]

Many moms call their babies by pet names or even just Baby. "Where's my baby? Or "Is baby hungry?" are commonly used phrases. Compare those with the phrases, "Where's (baby's name)? Or "Is (baby's name) hungry?"

Many babies learn to recognize their names between four and six months. If you want to help your child learn their name, call them by name frequently. While we all call our babies Baby at times, using their given names more often is an easy habit to form. Pet names are also acceptable and common in all cultures.

Babies typically understand words and simple phrases many months before they can say them. Using your child's name during the day will help them recognize it. Baby development experts recommend you narrate your day, so your child learns words and language. Some moms feel strange telling their babies what they're doing, such as "Mommy sees (baby's name)!" Make it your goal to do a bit more than you prefer. Some mothers talk a lot, and others not so much. Be yourself but realize that the more you talk, the richer the language environment will be for your child.

Ways to Encourage Your Baby's Development:

- Frequently spend time talking to each other face-to-face. What you talk about doesn't matter much; however, babies don't need to hear your burdens and should never hear that they are one.
- Play "Where's (baby's name)?" Hide from your baby and ask, "Where's (baby's name)?" Gain your child's attention, then pop up from behind the sofa or underneath the covers as you say, "There you are!" Most kids love this variation of the peekaboo game.

Things to Remember:

I'll schedule your six-month-old baby pictures.
If your baby doesn't respond when you call, make sure they can hear. Frequent ear infections and allergies can cause fluid in the ears that muffle sounds.

Chapter 68

Lazy Baby

It seems daft to call a child lazy simply because he or she hasn't yet developed the physical strength or skill to cross a room on their own.[1]

No mother wants her baby to struggle or have delays in development. But when she notices that her child isn't doing what other babies are doing, she can't help but wonder if something is wrong. Most of us question whether we've been negligent or are to blame. Thoughts arise like *Maybe I shouldn't have done _______when I was pregnant* or *What am I doing wrong?* Moms often blame themselves even when they may not be responsible.

I wish parents were never responsible for a child's disability. But sometimes they are. Child abuse, drug abuse during pregnancy, and maternal neglect frequently happen. However, delays also occur in children who have ideal parents and loving environments.

When a child isn't meeting a milestone, most of the time there's a reason. If your baby isn't yet sitting up or holding their bottle, laziness isn't the cause. Your baby may have low muscle tone or weakness that makes these activities exhausting or impossible. They may have motor coordination difficulties that make it hard to achieve these seemingly easy-to-meet milestones. Whatever the case, laziness isn't one of the reasons.

Words matter and labels stick. Never have I met anyone who wanted to be called lazy. I'm not a gambler, but if I were, I'd wager that your baby wouldn't like to be called lazy either, especially when they're doing their best.

Ways to Encourage Your Baby's Development:

- Praise your baby's efforts. For example, "I see you're trying hard to hold your bottle." All of us work harder for praise, even babies.
- Some babies don't achieve milestones because they lack enough opportunities to practice. Therefore, offer your baby many opportunities during the day to work on their play skills.

Things to Remember:

I won't ever call you lazy, and I won't allow others to do that either.
I'll make a daily schedule so you get frequent opportunities to practice.

Chapter 69

Can't Lie Down

90% of parenting is just thinking about
when you can lie down again.[1]

Your baby will soon learn how to sit up by themselves. However, getting back down from that position without falling and getting hurt will take a few more months. In the meantime, your child will topple over hundreds of times before they master sitting and playing without losing their balance.

As your child gains these new mobility skills, your heart bursts with pride. However, your brain and body also become exhausted because your mommy radar constantly alerts you to danger.

When I read the above quote, I laughed. When my babies were young, I daydreamed about lying down to rest in that carefree way I enjoyed before kids. Have you thought that as well?

One thing that also blocked my ability to rest was I couldn't lay down my fears. Since I worked at the children's hospital, I treated children who had suffered injuries from often-preventable accidents. As a result, preventing a preventable accident became an obsession, one that exhausted me.

If you're also a worrier, accept that you have an issue with control. I learned that while I could protect my child most of the time, accidents still happened. Learn to delegate supervision of your baby to those you trust. While they may do things a little differently than you, your baby needs you for the long haul. Depression, anger, and hopelessness can arise when you exhaust yourself.

To prevent becoming overwhelmed, give some of your responsibilities to others and rest. Fifteen minutes is better than nothing. Start small and gain confidence that your baby will be fine.

Ways to Encourage Your Baby's Development:

- Continue placing pillows around your baby while they sit on the floor. Always supervise your baby to prevent injury.
- Grandparents or trusted friends are great options so you can rest. In addition, babies benefit from getting used to different people.

Things to Remember:

I'll schedule regular time to rest.
I'll keep a cold pack in the freezer to soothe my baby when they bump their head.

Chapter 70

Pureed Foods

By 4 months to 6 months, most babies are ready to begin eating solid foods as a complement to breast-feeding or formula-feeding.[1]

While your baby still gets most of their nourishment from either breastmilk or formula, most babies can begin pureed foods around this time. Consult your child's doctor to see if they feel your baby is ready to eat solids.

Here are some signs that your tot is ready. Your baby will have steady head control when upright. Good head control indicates your baby's neck muscles are strong enough to assist with swallowing semi-solid foods. There are numerous muscles that perform swallowing, and many are in the face and neck.

Your baby will also be able to sit without support. While they aren't yet sitting on their own, they should be steady, not wobbly, in the upright position. Again, sitting steady indicates neck and trunk strength, which are needed to safely eat solid foods.

Follow your doctor's instructions on what foods to begin with and how to progress. Always have your child seated during feedings, and don't force your baby to eat foods they refuse. Offer an item and see what happens. If they act disinterested, spit it out, or throw up, discontinue that food for a while. You can always try again in a few days. If problems persist, talk with the doctor.

Eating should be a pleasant experience. Therefore, allow your baby to lead and don't make it a battle. You don't want them to think eating solid food is unpleasant.

Ways to Encourage Your Baby's Development:

- Follow your doctor's recommendations on beginning pureed foods. Start slow with small portions.
- Food preferences will change over time. Expect it. Allow your baby to touch and explore foods to increase their tolerance of the smells and textures.

Things to Remember:

I expect you to get messy when you eat.
Your favorite food right now is

______________________________________.

Chapter 71

Where's Baby?

Today's goal: keep the tiny humans alive.[1]

Many years ago, I treated a baby who had Down Syndrome. He had the typical low muscle tone and lack of energy to move around that many babies with this diagnosis have. For months, his mother and I had worked on strengthening and encouraging him to roll over. At times I was unsure if he'd ever learn to roll. While his mother remained hopeful, she was discouraged.

One day when they arrived for his appointment, his mom had a story to share. She had laid her child on the floor mat in the living room, as she usually did, and had gone into the kitchen to prepare dinner. After a few moments, she realized she wasn't hearing any sounds from the other room. She peeked around the corner, and her baby was gone.

She had left him playing on the floor mat. *Where is he?* she wondered as she frantically searched the room. Eventually, she peeked underneath the sofa, and there he was. Her son never babbled or cried very much, so when she saw him among the dust bunnies, he was content but stuck.

Finally, her baby boy had rolled over. Apparently, he had rolled over a few times and got stuck underneath the couch. While mom was ecstatic that her son had finally rolled, she was overcome with fear when her baby disappeared. Expect your baby to do the unexpected. Luckily, this story turned out well, but that's not always the case. Never take your eyes off your child.

Ways to Encourage Your Baby's Development:

- Continue using a safe area on the floor or use a playpen so your baby can move around and not disappear underneath the furniture.
- Continue with the game "Where's baby?" by covering your tot's face with a cloth and asking, "Where's baby?" Use an excited tone of voice. Encourage your baby to reach up and pull the cloth off their face. When they do, joyfully say, "There you are!"

Things to Remember:

You love pulling the cloth off your face.
I'll buy foam mats for the floor area where you play.

Chapter 72

Don't Drop That

Around 6 months old, babies start to delightfully drop objects—on purpose. This can be annoying for parents but it's actually important for tots to do.[1]

Has your baby started dropping things on purpose? When your child was younger, dropping things was accidental. By now, the dropping should be intentional. You may even notice your child watching the item fall.

When your patience wears thin, remind yourself this too shall pass. They aren't doing this activity to annoy you. On the contrary, they enjoy watching things fall and bounce on the floor. Since you're an adult, you know the dropped items have to be picked up. However, your baby is mastering an essential cognitive skill.

As babies grow, most moms know to check their child's motor and feeding development. For example, we know when our babies should be sitting up or when to start feeding them baby food. But we're not as aware of cognitive development. Children's "thinking skills" are measured by how they play with their toys. Dropping items on purpose and watching to see where they go are signs of cognitive advancement.

Yay! Your baby is making up games. Take a deep breath and smile, because this messy phase will pass one day. In the meantime, at least the pets love it.

Ways to Encourage Your Baby's Development:

- Continue dropping blocks into a container, then encourage your baby to drop blocks into it too. Now that they're dropping things on purpose, show them where to drop the item.
- When they drop an item, ask, "Where did it go?" Pick it up and show them, saying, "Here it is!" You don't have to do this every time. Mix it up so both of you enjoy the game.

Things to Remember:

You love to drop your

____.

You began dropping items on purpose on

______________________________.

Chapter 73

Oh No!

Between 6 and 11 months of age, your baby should learn to understand the word no and will stop what he is doing (although he may immediately do it again!)[1]

When your baby is midway through his first year, they begin to understand the word *no*. Since they're young and not getting into too much danger, they may have rarely heard the word. But with more mobility and exploration, they'll hear it a lot. Some parents joke that their child hears the word *no* so many times that they believe their name is No.

Shaking the head to indicate no is a gesture babies learn early. You can shake your head while you say no to teach your child what both the gesture and word mean. If you wag your finger while saying no, don't be surprised if, one day, your child wags their finger back at you. Babies mimic what they see.

When you play with your baby, drop an item in a bucket and say, "Oh no!" When your baby drops an object into it, say, "Oh no!" Your child may giggle and want to repeat the action. To add to the giggles, place your hands on your cheeks as Macaulay Culkin did in the movie *Home Alone*. Babies love facial expressions!

Oh No!

Ways to Encourage Your Baby's Development:

- The word *no* is a crucial safety word your child needs to learn. We automatically say it with a firmer tone to gain attention.
- Sing songs to help your baby transition to another toy when you tire of the drop-it-and-mommy-picks-it-up game.

Things to Remember:

You first shook your head no on

____.

It is typical for babies to respond differently to a dad's deeper voice than to a mom's higher pitch.

Chapter 74

Blowing Raspberries

Babies start blowing raspberries, which look like a cluster of tiny spit bubbles, between 4 and 7 months old. It's one of the ways they develop language skills.[1]

As your baby begins teething, they may also start blowing spit bubbles. This behavior is called blowing raspberries. Babies in all cultures do it. You can play with your child by blowing raspberries back and forth, and you may both laugh.

While making raspberry sounds, your baby is learning to purse their lips and blow air out of their mouth. These are essential skills as your baby begins to figure out how to communicate in ways other than crying or fussing.

Dads love to blow raspberries on their baby's belly because giggles often result. Moms love it too, but daddies often enjoy the physical play more. You can also see if your baby will blow raspberries on your arms or belly. Motor imitation is the way your baby soaks up knowledge during this phase of life. Making funny sounds, like blowing raspberries, often gets babies' attention, and they love it.

Another fun way to encourage your baby to make sounds is to lightly pat your hand on your child's mouth while they are cooing. The sound created is one which most babies enjoy. You can do this to yourself, then to your baby. These fun baby games help your child learn valuable skills that eventually lead to talking.

Ways to Encourage Your Baby's Development:

- When your baby coos, lightly pat your hand repeatedly over their mouth, so it makes a funny sound. You can also do this in front of a mirror for added fun.
- While your child coos, take their hand and lightly pat it on their mouth. Doing this teaches them how to make the sounds by themselves.

Things to Remember:

You began blowing raspberries on

____.

Your first tooth came in on

____.

Chapter 75

Sleeping All Night

Babies between 4 and 6 months old are developmentally able to sleep through the night without feeding, but whether they do is another story. Babies, like adults, eat for comfort and pleasure, not just nourishment.[1]

When your baby begins sleeping through the night, you may feel like you've died and gone to heaven. For many mothers, the first time this happens, they panic, thinking something's wrong because their baby didn't cry at night. However, after they realize everything is fine, they may allow themselves to dream about a future where they finally get enough sleep.

While most babies can sleep six to eight hours without eating by four to six months, many don't. Why? Often the baby seeks comfort from the mom. At this age, nursing or feeding throughout the night may not be because the baby is hungry, although it's hard to tell.

Getting enough restful sleep is helpful for both you and your baby's health. During these months, make adjustments to help your baby learn how to self-soothe. For example, let them fuss or cry a little longer each time before patting their back or picking them up. The easiest time to begin these changes is during naps if those are also difficult. Continue working toward getting them used to your coming, but they must wait a bit. The goal is for them to go back to sleep while they wait and to realize they're okay.

Yes, this strategy is difficult for most mothers. But your child needs to learn how to self-soothe, knowing mom will come eventually.

WAYS TO ENCOURAGE YOUR BABY'S DEVELOPMENT:

- When your baby awakens from sleep, wait a little longer each time before going to help. Wait fifteen seconds the first time and thirty seconds the second. Keep doubling the time and see how that goes.
- Try talking to your baby without touching them if they awaken at night. If they feel your hand, they may always want cuddles. Self-soothing is a skill your baby needs to learn.

THINGS TO REMEMBER:

The first time you slept all night was

____.

When I check on you at night, I won't turn on the lights because that will make it harder for you to go back to sleep.

Chapter 76

Waving Bye-Bye

Waving is one of your baby's earliest forms of social communication.[1]

Babies are adorable when they wave bye-bye. While most babies won't wave until around eight months, go ahead and encourage yours to do so by waving bye-bye to them. For example, when daddy leaves for work, say bye-bye and wave while your baby watches. You can take your little one's hand and wave it, so they feel the motion.

Children learn what they hear and see, so model waving now. Make it fun by waving bye-bye as you put the toys away. "Bye-bye, toy." Or, when it is time for bed, they can wave bye-bye to everyone in the house and even to their favorite toys. When your child gets older and you want to wean them from the bottle, wave and say bye-bye to the bottle as you put it away. By now, your child should understand the bottle isn't permanently gone.

Typically, babies will wave bye before hi. These gestures are necessary forms of communication and social development. Distractions in the home, such as constant television noise, can cause your child to ignore others entering and leaving the room. To encourage more social engagement between your baby and the others in the home, minimize background noise as much as possible.

Waving bye-bye isn't merely a motor action. It's also a basic form of social engagement and communication. After all, everyone loves knowing someone cares enough about them to wave bye-bye. Showing your baby how to care about others is a primary role for parents. When your little one waves, it shows you they care that you're departing for a while.

Ways to Encourage Your Baby's Development:

- When you put your baby to bed at night, encourage them to wave bye-bye to others in the home.
- Play with your child face-to-face each day. Allowing your tot to play as they choose without ever interacting with others is unwise.

Things to Remember:

My favorite outfit on you right now is

____.

I'll schedule a few minutes to play face-to-face with you each day.

Chapter 77

Pushing Up

Using their arms to push up helps your baby prepare to roll over from their tummy to their back. This push-up position also strengthens your baby's upper body muscles, which are important for sitting up, crawling, and walking.[1]

By four months, most babies are pushing up on their forearms from their tummies. Some children learn how to do this earlier and others later. Babies who dislike playing on their stomachs may not learn how to push up on their arms or hands and miss the opportunity to develop strong arms and shoulders.

While discontinuing tummy-time play may seem insignificant, serious developmental risks can occur. For example, many babies who avoid tummy time can't push up and roll. Others will use their legs or lower body to flip themselves onto their backs. While it's good these babies can roll from their tummy to their back, performing the motion without pushing up on their arms may slow future skills development.

Some milestones that require strong arms and hands are holding spoons, manipulating switches, climbing playground equipment, and riding a tricycle. The foundation for these skills is the simple activity of pushing up onto arms and hands from the tummy.

Pushing Up

If your baby continues to struggle with pushing up onto their arms and hands after four months, talk with your child's doctor. A developmental assessment may help you discover ways to make your baby comfortable with this important milestone.

Ways to Encourage Your Baby's Development:

- If your baby hates tummy time, try laying your child on your chest while you recline. You can also prop them up on their elbows and keep them entertained for a few minutes.
- Many babies fuss during tummy time. However, there's a difference between fussing and panic. Don't make your baby panicky. Unless your baby is panicking or vomiting, some fussing is common. Ask your child's doctor if you have concerns.

Things to Remember:

You began pushing up onto your forearms on

____.

I'll prop you on your forearms and encourage you to stay there for a few minutes.

Chapter 78

Going for a Ride

What is it about a car ride that seems to cast a spell on a wide-awake baby?[1]

When your baby fusses and cries and won't go to sleep, most moms get desperate. Walking, rocking, and bouncing work sometimes. But other times sleep struggles can only be solved by going for a ride in the car. For example, when my babies were younger, we drove around in the neighborhood many nights. My son slept like a champ while the car quietly meandered through the neighborhood. But the minute we stopped, he woke up.

A scientific explanation for this common phenomenon may exist. When your baby is going for a ride in the car, they are in a safe, warm, quiet environment, like being in the womb. The moving vehicle makes sounds and motions that help your baby relax. Plus, the inside of most cars is pretty dull, and sleep ensues when your tot has nothing to do.

Our bodies have a vestibular system that responds to movement. Rapid motions, such as falling, make us alert and aware of the danger; however, gentle, rhythmic ones soothe us. We know this automatically because when our babies fuss, we gently rock and sway them. The motion of riding in the car feels similar. Plus, the engine's humming adds white noise, blocking other sounds that may keep your baby awake.

Have you taken your baby for rides in the car to get them to sleep? If not, give it a try, because sometimes it may be the only way that works. But, of course, that means you don't get to sleep.

Ways to Encourage Your Baby's Development:

- Going for a ride in the car or stroller can relax your baby so they'll sleep. Sleep is essential for healthy growth and development.
- Maintain regular nap and sleep schedules. Unfortunately, sleep schedules get thrown off when your baby is sick or teething. When your baby is better, work toward returning to the regular schedule.

Things to Remember:

When you ride in the car, most often you will

____.

After dinner, I'll take you for an evening stroll to help you sleep better.

Chapter 79

Having a Ball

The humble ball was inducted into the US National Toy Hall of Fame in 2009. But its role in childhood play stretches back to the beginnings of civilization.[1]

Babies love balls, and this has apparently been true since the beginning of time. Ancient Egyptian ruins show children played with balls made from papyrus or leather stuffed with straw. Balls are a cause-and-effect toy offering your child endless fun. Picking it up and dropping it on the floor is a fascinating game. Watching the ball bounce and roll around gives your child practice tracking the ball's movements with their eyes.

When your baby can sit up, rolling a ball back and forth is a social event they'll enjoy. Getting down on the floor and facing your child is the kind of engagement that builds relationships. Watching two cartoon characters on a screen rolling a ball back and forth may be funny to your child, but it won't teach them the game or improve their eye-hand coordination and visual tracking skills.

Your baby needs good eye-hand coordination and visual tracking for upcoming schoolwork, such as handwriting, cutting, and pasting. Some believe you only need good eye-hand coordination for sports.

Yes, for many sports, those skills are required. But schoolwork also challenges your child's abilities to write neatly and cut on a line. Both require visual and eye-hand coordination skills. Who knew such a simple thing as rolling a ball back and forth with your baby could impact their future academic abilities?

Ways to Encourage Your Baby's Development:

- At this early age, your baby won't be able to roll the ball back to you, but it's still fun and helpful for them to try.
- Offer different balls of various sizes and textures to enhance your baby's experiences.

Things to Remember:

Your favorite ball to play with is

____.

I'll ask others to play ball with you in the evenings while I cook dinner.

Chapter 80

Small Talk

The very best "toy" for your young child is you.[1]

What do you talk to your baby about? Anything. You can talk about the weather, how beautiful their smile is, or what you're cooking for dinner. When they coo or babble, return those sounds to encourage more. Think of it as small talk. When you attend social functions, small talk or cocktail conversation is an art. Everyone knows to avoid politics or religion. Instead, you keep it light and talk about a movie or a vacation.

The same goes for your baby. They don't need to hear about divisive topics or overhear arguments. Keep it light. Talk about how much you love fun activities. Television shows or screen-based activities don't improve interactive communication skills, even though your child is mesmerized by them.

Passive watching isn't the same as engaging in a back-and-forth conversation, even if it's nothing but babbling. Also, background television or handheld screen noise can interfere with your baby's focus on what you're saying and minimize eye contact. Consider turning off those devices, replacing them with music or silence.

It may take some time to adjust to turning off your favorite shows, but these days of your baby's life pass quickly. A lot of learning occurs every day, and your baby's brain is soaking up sounds and words. So, fill their world with good words—ones that convey "I love you, and you are important."

WAYS TO ENCOURAGE YOUR BABY'S DEVELOPMENT:

- Sing silly songs during the day. Make up your own if you want.
- Tell them you love them throughout the day.

THINGS TO REMEMBER:

Read short books to your baby during the day.
One book I want to read to you is
____.

Section Three

Seven To Nine Months

Chapter 81

Stranger Danger

Stranger anxiety is a normal emotional phase that occurs when your child cries or becomes distressed when an unknown person approaches or attempts to hold her.[1]

During this phase of your baby's development, they're learning that when an object goes away, it's not only gone, but they miss it. While they may cry when their bottle drops out of reach, they scream when mommy leaves—even if it's only for a moment. This phase is tough for moms.

Your child knows their people—those in their world who are familiar. When they cry, you know they prefer that their folks remain nearby where they can see them. During these months, they're also learning to spot unfamiliar people, even ones they used to love, such as grandparents, aunts, or uncles. While it often upsets those familiar now unfamiliar-to-baby people, this phase is typical. And it *is* a phase. As with the earlier stages of your baby's development, this too shall pass.

In the meantime, don't shame or force your child to go to unfamiliar people, even family members, if they're upset. Although it's okay to encourage them to let grandma hold them, don't force them if they're overwrought with fear. As with all skills, babies learn them at their own pace. Be patient.

WAYS TO ENCOURAGE YOUR BABY'S DEVELOPMENT:

- Sit beside the unfamiliar-to-baby family member with your child in your lap. See if they tolerate sitting near the person. Move farther away if they're too afraid but continue to visit with the person and remain calm. Hopefully, your baby will pick up from your cues that this person is safe.
- Don't shame your baby for being afraid of people they should be okay with. Never call them names or get angry because they feel unsafe. Instead say, "I see you're afraid. Everything's okay."

THINGS TO REMEMBER:

The people you will no longer go to are

____.

When we go shopping, strangers seem to make you

____.

Chapter 82

Want a Cracker?

When it comes to baby teeth eruption, there's a wide range of normal. The average first baby tooth erupts at 6 or 7 months, but first teeth may emerge at around 12 months old (or even later).[1]

The teething process seems to last a long time. Some children hardly fuss as their teeth come in, while others cry and fuss day and night. Your child may already have a tooth because some babies are even born with a few incisors, and others have one by three or four months. Either way, your baby is probably chewing on everything, including you.

When teething begins, many moms start offering their tots teething crackers or other foods that quickly dissolve. You may also want to give your baby something safe to chew. Soft, rubber teething rings are easy for your baby to hold. If your little one can sit in the highchair, place safe teething toys or crackers on the tray for them to pick up and gnaw.

As always, never leave your baby unattended. Keep your attention on them at all times. Even though those teething biscuits are soft and shouldn't cause choking, accidents happen and happen fast. Your tot may bite off too big a piece while you're at the front door retrieving a package. You may only be gone a minute, but that minute is all it takes for your baby to choke.

Double-check with your doctor if you have concerns about whether your baby is ready for baby crackers or teething biscuits. Never feed your child anything unless they're sitting upright and you're watching them constantly. If your baby continually pushes food out of their mouth, gags excessively, or vomits, talk with the doctor. An assessment may provide answers and ways to help your baby begin to enjoy foods and eat.

Ways to Encourage Your Baby's Development:

- Offer your baby the biscuit and see if they reach for it. If not, place it in their hand to hold. Next, you can say, "Do you want a cracker?" or "Are your gums hurting?" Hearing these phrases enriches your baby's vocabulary.
- If your baby doesn't have steady head control or has struggled with sucking and swallowing from a bottle, proceed slowly and with caution. Make sure your doctor is okay with your baby trying soft foods.

Things to Remember:

You have _____ teeth.
I'll buy some soft teething rings or other safe toys you can chew.

Chapter 83

That's Heavy

Yay! It's the weekend! Oh wait, I'm a mum.[1]

By the latter half of your baby's first year, they should be using both hands together. For example, they may hold two toys and bang them together or try to pick up a heavy, bulky toy using both hands. Using their hands in concert to get something is a positive development in your baby's life.

A fun way to encourage your little one to pick up bigger toys while making sounds is to grunt when you pick up a toy. Does your baby imitate your actions? Or you can say, "That's heavy!" as you pick up something. Pairing appropriate words with the activity teaches your baby verbs. Most of us teach nouns or labels for objects but forget to use action words or descriptors frequently. For example, we label items such as cups or bottles. However, we don't often say, "[Child's name] is drinking from a bottle."

Again, babies of this age are moving and exploring, so they have numerous opportunities to grunt as they struggle to pick up something or push you away. Grunting isn't only a typical vocalization for babies, but it also strengthens your child's diaphragm muscle. That muscle is vital for mobility and talking. So, have fun with your baby by grunting and exclaiming how heavy something is. And again, be exaggerated and expressive so they pay attention.

WAYS TO ENCOURAGE YOUR BABY'S DEVELOPMENT:

- Large, soft blocks are appropriate toys for your baby to pick up with both hands.
- Model using both of your hands to pick up a block while saying, "This block is heavy!" You may also grunt and moan in playful ways. Babies often love these types of interactions.

THINGS TO REMEMBER:

I'll buy some big, soft blocks for you.
You began picking up larger toys using both hands on

______________________________.

Chapter 84

Dada

Cross cultural research on baby's first words shows that the clear winner is Dada.[1]

Most babies are babbling by now. While you wish mama was your child's first word, it's probably dada. While a child of this young age is merely babbling dada, it still stings. Since moms are often the primary caretaker, most are at least a little annoyed that the child calls first for dada, not mama.

As speech experts attempt to uncover why babies say dada first, they remain undecided about the reason. Could the *d* sound be easier for babies to pronounce than the *m* sound? Maybe. But some babies babble mama first or even other names, like papa. So, for those children, why would they say a more difficult consonant first? Currently, science has no concrete answers.

Regardless, mamas don't like it. Some experts think babies call for dada first because daddies are often the parent who leaves the house most, and the child is calling for him. Who knows. Anyway, rest easy: babbling speech—whether dada or mama—isn't intentional language. In other words, your baby isn't specifically calling for daddy or mommy. That skill comes later. While it stings for your child not to call you mama, take comfort in your baby's burgeoning communication skills.

At this age, encourage more talking by repeating back to them whatever sounds your baby makes. Also, look for your baby to gain two or three other consonant-vowel combinations over the upcoming months, such as papa or mama. And even if they don't, keep talking to them. Babies listen and learn for a long time before they begin talking.

WAYS TO ENCOURAGE YOUR BABY'S DEVELOPMENT:

- When baby babbles dadada, bababa, mamama, or whatever, repeat it and act interested in the "conversation."
- Babble to each other while looking in a mirror. Babies watch how we move our mouths, which helps them learn how to say words.

THINGS TO REMEMBER:

Your first word was

____.

You said it on

____.

Chapter 85

Say Mama!

Mom: One who sacrifices her body, sleep, social life, spending money, eating hot meals, peeing alone, patience, energy and sanity for love.[1]

Every mother wants her baby to call her Mama. When your child calls you Mama, it feels like they know you. With that one word, they've shown you're their mother and they need you. Mothers of children who don't call them Mama or those whose baby seems not to notice them often struggle. Mamas do a lot to care for their babies, and most don't ask for much. But each wants to be loved and recognized for what she does. That simple name, *Mama*, goes a long way in giving her the attachment she craves.

If your baby isn't calling you Mama, encourage them to say it by calling yourself Mama. For example, if your baby wants a bottle, say, "Mama will get it." Daddy can help by playing a game called "Where's Mama?" In this version of peekaboo, mama hides and daddy carries the baby around the house calling, "Where's Mama?" First, they look behind a door. "Is she in here? No, Mama's not in here." Daddy and baby continue moving around the house, looking behind doors and around corners until they find her. Daddy then says, "There's Mama!"

Say Mama!

Babies learn the words they hear repeatedly. So, call yourself Mama during your day, so they hear it and identify you as Mama.

Ways to Encourage Your Baby's Development:

- Get face-to-face with your baby and say, "Mama." You can place your baby's hand on your mouth as you vocalize the word so they can feel the vibrations of your mouth.
- Make sure your baby can get their lips together to form the *m* sound. Talk to your baby's doctor if they can't.

Things to Remember:

The first time you called me Mama was on

____.

I'll talk to the doctor if you're not yet saying the word *mama*.

Chapter 86

Open and Close

Your baby will love it if you can dedicate a cupboard or drawer in the spaces you often spend time in.[1]

Your baby may now enjoy picking things up and dropping them repeatedly. They also may have discovered drawers and cabinet doors. And once they learn how to jerk them open and slam them shut, watch out. They'll open and close and open and close them over and over. Then they'll pull out whatever objects are in the drawer. Naturally, you'll get frustrated, whether the cabinet is full of socks, underwear, or old movies. There's also your dismay at finding your muffin pans, cookie sheets, plastic containers, and dish towels scattered across your kitchen floor. Oh my!

Opening and closing drawers or doors is another example of cause-and-effect play. Learning this cognitive skill, where your baby does something and observes the result, is vital. But you ask, "Why does it take so long for them to learn?" We adults make some of the same mistakes over and over. We then ask ourselves, "Why haven't I learned that yet?" And speaking for myself, some lessons I've never learned.

During this phase of your child's development, dedicate a drawer or cabinet your baby can safely explore. Ensure the furniture your baby is playing with won't fall on your child. Expect the unexpected. Your child may decide to climb in the drawer or yank it hard. Fill the low cabinet or drawer with baby-safe everyday household objects, such as wooden spoons, plastic containers and cups, and toys.

Allow your baby to play in their cabinet. If they want to get into the other ones—and they will—gently redirect them back to their area. If you don't want your ears to hurt from the incessant banging, don't offer them metal pots and pans.

Ways to Encourage Your Baby's Development:

- Babies routinely choose to explore everyday objects over toys. So, offer plastic measuring cups, wooden spoons, remote controls with batteries removed, and clean hairbrushes or toothbrushes.
- Make sure your baby can't pinch their fingers when they close the drawer or door. Always keep your other drawers and lower cabinets safely off limits by installing locks.

Things to Remember:

Your favorite household object to explore is

____.

I'll purchase some cabinet locks for the other cabinets you aren't free to explore.

Chapter 87

Combat Crawling

Babies usually start crawling when they are between 7 and 12 months old.[1]

After sitting, parents begin anticipating crawling as their child's next significant milestone. Unfortunately, crawling can be delayed or skipped for many babies who haven't enjoyed much tummy time. If your child doesn't crawl, that doesn't mean they won't walk. However, babies who crawl have stronger arms and core muscles than those who don't crawl.

The combat crawl is the first forward motion most babies learn. While rolling is also a form of mobility, your baby can't wiggle forward while rolling. Now that your child can scooch or crawl on the belly, they can finally slink under the chair or through a tunnel.

Your baby is getting ready to combat crawl when they can prop on one elbow and reach forward with the other arm when on their tummy. Some babies prefer to scoot or combat crawl backward. While these motions are good, forward movement is ideal. You want your baby to have the strength to propel their body forward because that motion is more complex and requires more force than pushing backward.

Combat Crawling

Some mothers say, "My baby is smart enough to do things the easy way." However, while the child is doing their best, crawling backward won't help them eventually crawl on hands and knees or walk. Both of those skills require significant strength and coordination, and combat crawling backward doesn't adequately strengthen them. To summarize, crawling backward is better than not doing so, but forward crawling is preferred.

Ways to Encourage Your Baby's Development:

- Provide plenty of time on the floor for your baby to figure out how to crawl. Trial and error are how this usually occurs, so lots of practice is needed.
- When your baby plays on the floor, place toys slightly out of reach to encourage crawling toward them.

Things to Remember:

The first time you combat crawled was on

____.

I'll create a larger safe zone on the floor where you can play.

Chapter 88

W-Sitting

If they do it for long periods of time, it can cause problems with physical development.[1]

You may ask yourself, "Is my baby sitting in a W-sitting position?" Here's how to check: When your child sits on the floor, stand in front of them and look down. If your baby's legs form the letter W (legs bent at the knees, feet back near the hips), you have a W-sitter. Ideally, your baby should sit with their legs relaxed in front of them, not splayed out to either side.

Babies should be able to sit on the floor with their legs in various positions, especially by age nine to ten months. However, when your child sits exclusively in the W-sitting position, some possible problems may arise. All of them are undesirable.

The W-sitting position prevents your baby from developing strong muscles in the hip and core because when the legs are splayed, your child can't fall over. Their legs prevent a sideways fall. Therefore, your baby doesn't use their core muscles to prevent a fall. When those muscles remain weak, the result may be poor walking balance.

The W-sitting position also places pressure on your baby's hip and knee joints, often leading to deformity. Some babies will develop leg deformity and pain, which can impact them when they're older. Neither of these conditions is repairable without orthopedic surgery, so prevention in the early years is the best advice.

Ways to Encourage Your Baby's Development:

- Sit on the floor with your baby and reposition their legs out of the W-sitting position. Keep them engaged with toys or books, so they learn to sit in new ways longer.
- If your baby doesn't tolerate moving both legs out of the W-sitting position, only reposition one leg. Next time, change places with the other one. Some alteration is better than none.

Things to Remember:

I'll talk to the doctor about your constant W-sitting.
Your favorite book right now is

____.

Chapter 89

Steady Sitting

At the end of 7 months, your baby should be able to sit unsupported. If this milestone isn't met, check in with your physician.[1]

When your baby can sit steadily on the floor, you can breathe a sigh of relief. Now, you can allow your child to sit and play, freeing you up to do other tasks while still keeping a close eye on them. Placing some cushions nearby can prevent injury from a hard fall.

While many babies learn to sit steadily by seven months, not all do. Some take a little longer, and if your baby was born prematurely, use the adjusted age to decide how your tot is progressing. If your baby is still falling forward or propping on their arms, continue working on sitting and talk to your child's doctor.

Steady sitting demonstrates that your baby's core muscles are strong, and they can now move a little bit without falling. They should eventually try to get back down by themselves and may even be moving from their belly to a sitting position. Most babies, however, take a little longer to learn these movements.

Using baby seats for the floor, such as a Bumbo, won't advance your little one's sitting skills as much as you think. These baby-holding devices prevent falls and offer another place for the baby to play, but they don't strengthen the muscles your baby needs to use to sit on their own. So, if you use such seats, do so sparingly.

Ways to Encourage Your Baby's Development:

- Provide multiple daily opportunities for your baby to practice sitting on the floor.
- Keep toys your baby enjoys nearby. For example, pop-up toys are entertaining and age appropriate. Picking up rattles and putting them in a container are also developmentally helpful.

Things to Remember:

You first sat steadily by yourself on

______________________________________.

I'll buy a pop-up toy that has different switches (buttons, slides, etc.) so you can learn how those work.

Chapter 90

Getting into Sitting

By 7 months, some babies may sit up from a lying-down position by pushing up from the stomach, but most little ones will need a grown-up pulling them up or placing them into a sitting position until around month 11.[1]

Limber babies may go from lying on their tummy to sitting up by placing their legs into a full split. Babies who aren't super flexible will push up onto their hands and knees and then sit on the side of their hip before moving into sitting.

Again, if you want your little one to learn how to get into a sitting position, they need lots of practice on the floor. As your baby becomes steadier in sitting, they may cry for you when they want to lie down. Instead of picking them up and then laying them down, guide them from sitting to lying on their belly. Doing this will allow them to feel how to accomplish the movement and help them learn to do it themselves.

The reverse is also true. When your child is on their tummy and wants to sit up, guide their body up to sitting without picking them up. You can add some fun by saying, "Baby up!" when helping them sit and "Baby down!" when assisting them to their tummy. Always strive to make the activity fun.

WAYS TO ENCOURAGE YOUR BABY'S DEVELOPMENT:

- To move your child from sitting on the floor to lying on their tummy, hold them around their ribs and gently guide them down. You may have to lean them slightly to the side to accomplish this.
- When your baby is on their tummy, hold them around the ribs and guide them up to a sitting position. Try not to allow them to put their legs into a split.

THINGS TO REMEMBER:

The first time you got into a sitting position from your tummy by yourself was on ____________________.
You can now sit steadily on the floor for ________________minutes.

Chapter 91

Sitting to Crawling

Babies typically start to crawl around the 9-month marker or later, but some start as early as 6 or 7 months, while others take their sweet time putting four on the floor. And some babies actually bypass crawling altogether—going straight from sitting up to standing to walking.[1]

Babies often learn to get on their hands and knees and rock back and forth in preparation for learning to crawl. Others push up from their bellies onto their hands and knees and then back into a sitting position. Later they'll learn to move from sitting to rocking on their hands and knees to crawling. These are typical patterns; however, other ways of movement also occur.

When babies can transition from one position to another, such as from sitting to crawling, new levels of independence are achieved. You know this automatically. They're more independent when they can safely change position from sitting to lying on their tummy, and you don't have to help. Yay!

For all these transitional movements, your baby must push up on their arms and hands. In previous chapters, I mentioned that a lack of adequate tummy time could result in delayed skills in the future, and this is one of those areas. If your little one refuses to push up onto their hands, how will they move from their tummy to sitting or sitting to crawling? Bearing weight on the hands is also essential for crawling on the hands and knees. So, keep doing the floor time and resist putting your baby in containers such as seats, standers, or jumpers. These baby-holding devices don't provide opportunities for your child to put weight on their hands.

Ways to Encourage Your Baby's Development:

- To help your baby get onto their hands and knees from sitting, hold them around the ribs and gently guide them. You may have to keep them in that position so they place some weight on their hands and knees.
- Sit on the floor and seat your child between your legs. Gently lay them over your straight leg so they're on their hands and knees. Your leg helps hold them there. Some children enjoy this position, which allows them to get used to balancing on their hands and knees.

Things to Remember:

The first time you got onto your hands and knees was on

______________________________.

I won't compare my child to other babies of the same age. Every baby is unique.

Chapter 92

Clapping Hands

Most babies are able to clap around 9 months, after they've mastered sitting up, pushing and pulling themselves up with their hands, and pre-crawling. (All that upper body strength helps them have the coordination to clap, too.)[1]

For months, you've wanted to know what your child is thinking. Maybe now you're getting a glimpse. Show them one of their favorite foods and ask, "Do you want this?" If they clap their hands and seem excited, they just said yes. While they didn't say the word *yes* or nod in acknowledgment, the gesture affirmed their answer.

Yay! Some important back-and-forth communication is occurring. Previously, your baby may have clapped their hands when you encouraged them to mimic your clapping motions. In the early months, clapping begins this way. The action has now progressed to the point where your baby understands and uses gestures as a form of language. They're communicating with intention.

You can test whether they genuinely understand the meaning of yes by offering them something you know they usually don't want. If they clap their hands in the same way, go ahead and give them the item and see what they do. If they toss it or fuss, you know their yes answer remains iffy.

As an evaluator for the local early intervention office, I interviewed many mothers whose heartfelt desire was to know what their baby wanted without having to guess all the time. If you feel that way, then you know the guessing game gets old, and both mom and baby often become frustrated. So, when your baby claps to say yes, be grateful your tot has met this critical milestone. To celebrate, clap your hands in delight.

Ways to Encourage Your Baby's Development:

- If your baby continues to need hand-over-hand help to make the clapping motion, keep doing it. For example, when you know they want an item, help them clap their hands and say, "Yes!" Then give them the item. Helping them clap yes before getting what they want will help them understand the connection.
- Hold up two items in front of your baby and ask, "Do you want the ______ or the _____?" See if they clap for what they want. Give them the one they indicated, so they learn to clap to communicate needs and wants.

Things to Remember:

The first day you clapped your hands to say yes was on

______________________________.

I'll talk to the doctor about

____.

Chapter 93

Let's Play Peekaboo

By months 9 to 12, your baby will likely be able to play peekaboo on her own.[1]

Most babies have learned the cognitive concept of object permanence by eight months. They know that when an object disappears out of sight, it isn't gone. For example, when your tot drops their pacifier, they search for it. They may look under their favorite blanket or around where they're sitting. When you dart out to the bathroom, they call for you because they know you're there even though you're not in sight.

So, now your little one may initiate playing peekaboo with you. They may lift the bib, cover their face, and then peek around to see you. Or they may hand you a blanket for you to cover your face so they can pull it off. While they aren't yet saying, "Peekaboo! I see you!" they delight when you do.

As discussed previously, peekaboo is a vital baby game that teaches cause and effect. In addition, peekaboo contains an important social engagement component that's missing from digital games. You and your baby are entertaining each other, and those moments are priceless.

Let's Play Peekaboo

While we all want our babies to have the best of everything and search for ideal toys and games, we often fall for the notion that the more expensive an item is, the better it must be. However, peekaboo can't be beaten among children's games that teach and build skills as well as meet developmental milestones. That's why peekaboo is a timeless and global activity. It can be played anywhere, at any time, and requires no equipment. Peekaboo is a winner!

Ways to Encourage Your Baby's Development:

- Cover your face with a blanket and encourage your baby to pull it off your face. Be excited when you say, "Peekaboo! I see you!" Add in a few tickles to boost the fun.
- If your baby is mobile, they may hide behind some furniture and peek out. When they do, yell, "Peekaboo! I see you!" Combining the game with movement is an effective way to help your baby engage with you and get moving.

Things to Remember:

The first time you initiated the peekaboo game was on

______________________________.

Your favorite game right now is

____.

Chapter 94

Baby on the Move

Infant walker-related injuries can be severe and can include skull fractures, brain injury, injuries to the face and neck, fractures to the arms and legs, burns, poisoning and drowning.[1]

When your baby begins crawling, either combat style or on hands and knees, the world becomes a more dangerous place. Unfortunately, accidents still happen even when you take every precaution you know to take, from blocking access to stairs to hiding electrical cords. Over the years of providing physical therapy to children, I've treated many kids injured in preventable accidents, such as nearly drowning in a few inches of water in a mop bucket to pulling down a hot iron onto themselves. So, as your baby begins to move around your home, you should expect the unexpected.

Baby walkers or other baby-holding equipment may seem like safe spots to park the baby while you do something else. You may leave the room or even go outside while watching your baby on a security camera, thinking all will be okay. However, if your baby manages to climb out and fall on their head, you'll watch the disaster unfold but won't be able to stop it.

I once treated a baby with a severe skull fracture who climbed out and fell from his play station. He hit his head on the edge of a brick hearth and was unconscious for days. No one thought that could happen; however, it did. He eventually woke up but continued to have seizures for a while. He had to relearn many skills he had previously mastered. But here's the kicker: a baby's future learning, such as academic performance in school, can be affected by childhood injuries like that one. Don't assume these accidents won't happen. Expect them. And do everything possible to avoid preventable accidents.

Ways to Encourage Your Baby's Development:

- Use baby gates and fencing to secure your baby's play area. Ensure no electrical cords, outlets, or sharp edges are present. Lock down everything.
- If you must leave the room, take your baby with you. Cameras allow you to watch your child but will not prevent serious injury if you're too far away.

Things to Remember:

I'll crawl around on the floor and see the area from your eye level, such as under furniture.

I'll be extra vigilant in picking up dropped coins and electronic batteries because my baby can quickly ingest those, and I may be unaware until it's too late.

Chapter 95

Getting into Stuff

The quickest way for a parent to get a child's attention is to sit down and look comfortable.[1]

Once your baby is on the move—either crawling or rolling—you'll wonder how they have so much energy and persistence to get into everything. Areas of your home that may have gone unnoticed for a while suddenly become a danger zone you never imagined. Those lovely baskets where you store odds and ends become your baby's obsession. Or maybe it's the drawer where you keep your video games or those candles in the fireplace. Yikes! Where are you going to put all this stuff so you can still enjoy them, but baby can't constantly dump them out or chew on them?

While there are no easy answers, I encourage you to put away anything dangerous to your baby. Yes, your life will be inconvenienced for a time, but this is only a phase. To illustrate why you should put things away, I'll share a true story. When I worked at the children's hospital, a baby who was an active crawler swallowed a hearing aid battery, also called a button battery. Unfortunately, no one saw it happen, and no one knew it occurred until the baby got sick.

He didn't choke on it, so no one suspected what the magnetic resonance imaging (MRI) would find. Imagine the horror and surprise when the results showed a small, round battery lodged in his throat, slowly leaking its toxic contents. Sadly, even though it was surgically removed, the chemicals that leaked from it had burned holes in the child's esophagus and trachea that couldn't be closed. As a result, he remained hospitalized for months while the holes closed on their own. He was placed in a medically induced coma, on a respirator, and fed through a tube to keep him quiet and allow healing to occur. All that horror occurred because of a hearing aid battery that went unnoticed by everyone except the baby.

Ways to Encourage Your Baby's Development:

- Frequently get down on the floor and look around. You may be surprised to find more danger than you imagined. Temporarily put away anything your baby shouldn't explore.
- Use a playpen when your baby needs to be mobile, and you can't watch them directly, such as during meal preparation or bathroom breaks.

Things to Remember:

The one item you're currently obsessed with getting into is

______________________________.

I'll buy more outlet covers and put away all breakables, including glass-top tables.

Chapter 96

Did You Call?

Most babies understand and respond to their own names by about 5 to 6 months of age, and most do by 9 months.[1]

Your baby's understanding of words (receptive language) develops earlier than their use of words (expressive language). This fact underlies my advice to talk to your baby a lot. The more they hear their name and the names of everyday items—such as bottle, ball, or binkie—the faster their understanding of language should advance.

During this phase of your baby's life, they may be turning when someone calls them. They may look to see who's talking or respond if they hear their older sibling yelling. They're aware of others and understand they should pay attention. If your child isn't turning when addressed or seems unaware when others are talking, make sure they can hear. Babies with allergies or chronic ear infections tend to build up fluid in their ears. This fluid muffles sounds and contributes to poor communication skills in those babies.

Earlier in the book, I shared the game called "Where's Mama?" You may recall this game teaches your baby that your name is Mama. You can modify that game and call it "Where's (your baby's name)?" Walk around where your child can see you and look under the cushions or behind furniture as you say, "Where's (your baby's name)?" When you see them, say, "There's (their name)!" Fun games like these help your baby learn their name.

Ways to Encourage Your Baby's Development:

- Play the "Where's (your baby's name)?" game and make it fun. Have other family members play as well. Older siblings or cousins love helping, so allow them to.
- Bang pots or shake keys behind your baby's head to see if they turn. Ensure they aren't distracted by other sounds, such as televisions or electronic tablets.

Things to Remember:

Playing "Where is ____?" games is a form of the peekaboo game, and babies love both versions.

You began turning when your name was called on

______________________________.

Chapter 97

Moving and Grooving

It's no secret that babies and toddlers love music—and playing tunes as well as dancing and listening to them are an important part of early child development.[1]

Your baby began listening to music in the womb. Now that they're older, maybe music is still a part of their day. Many moms keep some music playing, and some even change the playlist to include baby songs, such as traditional nursery rhymes. While classical sounds are recommended to be part of the musical menu, traditional nursery rhymes are timeless because they teach language concepts. Classical music is beneficial, as are nursery rhymes.

Simple rhythms paired with lyrics that contain lessons make learning enjoyable. Not all nursery rhymes have lessons, but some do. One of my all-time favorites is "The Wheels on the Bus." That song contains many motor actions your baby can learn. Learning motor actions now will help your baby imitate scribbling or get dressed one day. So, nursery rhymes with finger play prepare your baby to learn more practical uses of their hands and arms.

You have songs you love, so introduce your baby to a wide range of music. However, don't play music that includes curse words or language that demeans others. People need kindness, and our world won't become a kinder place unless each of us, and our children, do our part.

Ways to Encourage Your Baby's Development:

- Offer your baby rattles, pots, wooden spoons, or other ways to make sounds. Praise their efforts.
- If you're creative, write your own lyrics, using the music of a traditional nursery rhyme. Using songs to teach a routine, such as "time to eat," makes the activity more fun. Mary Poppins said, "A spoonful of sugar makes the medicine go down." Adding a fun element makes accomplishing a difficult task easier.

Things to Remember:

You're so cute when you wiggle to the song called

____.

Your favorite musical style seems to be

____.

Chapter 98

Don't Leave Me

I don't need a big, fancy vacation. I'd be happy with a trip to the bathroom by myself.[1]

Most babies will experience separation anxiety around nine months. One day your child plays happily while you briefly step away. The next day, they cry so hard that you'd think someone had cut off their leg. "I'm right here," you say repeatedly. But unless you pick them up and carry them around, they won't calm down.

While moms love knowing their babies want to be with them, these phases of separation anxiety can be frustrating. What seems like an overreaction to adults is the end of the world to your baby. You left!

Separation anxiety is a typical phase of your baby's development and will come and go for the first few years. As your child ages, new experiences with new people will challenge feelings of security. Don't get angry. Expect this response. Comfort your child with a calm voice and patience. However, don't let these anxious moments deter you from gradually introducing new experiences into your baby's life.

The more opportunities you provide for your child to be around other people both in and out of your home, the easier it should become for your tot to feel safe when you aren't constantly present.

Ways to Encourage Your Baby's Development:

- When your baby becomes fearful, calmly comfort them. Expect these phases and gently guide your child to try new experiences.
- Take regular trips to the park or schedule playdates with similarly aged children. Have cousins over to play. Refrain from cocooning your baby at home, as this will be counterproductive. Your baby's confidence will improve as they learn to feel okay during your absence and trust that mommy will return.

Things to Remember:

Your first episodes of separation anxiety appeared on

______________________________.

When you're around other children, you tend to

____.

Chapter 99

Pulling Off Socks

Babies take their socks off. All. The. Time.[1]

Why do babies constantly pull off their socks? Are they too hot? Do they dislike the sensation of wearing socks? Or are they simply exploring this new activity? I believe the answer is exploration. When babies discover how to reach their feet, they grab their toes and even put them in their mouths. So, if socks cover their feet, your baby simply grabs and pulls to see what happens.

That makes sense when viewed from a developmental perspective. But a busy, sleep-deprived mom becomes frustrated when her baby pulls off their socks for the millionth time. Or when she and the baby return to the car after a harried trip to the store and one sock is missing. It must be somewhere in the store. Ugh.

Just as babies learn to take toys apart or knock over block towers before they master putting things together or stacking blocks, the same is true with dressing. Your child will learn to take off clothes long before they know how to dress themselves. Socks are an example.

Many children are warmer than we are and can go barefoot without getting chilled. However, if your child does get cold, do what other mothers traditionally do. Dress your child in footed onesies so they can't undress their feet. When it comes to children, wise moms learn to outsmart them.

Ways to Encourage Your Baby's Development:

- If your baby struggles to reach their feet, dress them in socks with bells or balls attached. These objects will entice your child to reach and grab. However, don't allow your baby to swallow small items. Always keep a close eye on them.
- Keep reminding yourself that one day you want them to dress themselves. Learning how to undress comes first. Removing socks is part of the dressing process.

Things to Remember:

You ________________________ to wear socks.
Your favorite activity right now is

____.

Chapter 100

Timber!

It may look like your baby or toddler is simply destroying things or making a giant mess, but he is actually learning.[1]

You stack blocks into a tower, and your baby swats them down. An older playmate builds a fort using a sheet, and your child knocks it down. You ask, "Why are they tearing everything apart and making such a mess?" You may have even thought, *They're so destructive. What's wrong with them?*

Nothing is wrong; everything is correct. Babies of this age are in the deconstructing phase. Knocking things down, dumping them out, and scattering everything is how your baby learns what happens when they do specific actions. Putting the balls back into the bucket or stacking the blocks into a tower takes much more strength and coordination. Those skills come later.

In the meantime, have some fun with this phase. For example, when your baby knocks the tower over yell, "Timber!" Doing so is another example of a cause-and-effect game. This is your child's current phase of play. Making a mess is always easier, and more fun, than cleaning up. Even adults know that.

A game many dads enjoy is having the baby push them over as he yells, "Timber!" Active children love this, and it works off some of their excess energy. Dad loves it too. Roughhouse play is typical for children. Just ensure it doesn't get too rough and lead to injury.

Ways to Encourage Your Baby's Development:

- Stack throw pillows and have your baby knock them over by swatting or crawling into them.
- Children love surprises, and shouting "Timber!" pleases them. By the way, your child doesn't see a mess because they don't understand the concept yet.

Things to Remember:

You love knocking block towers over and dumping items out of containers.
I'll ask daddy or another family member to play with you in the evening before dinner, but we'll refrain from roughhousing before bed because we don't want to overstimulate you.

Chapter 101

For Me?

Tearing paper actually helps children develop so many essential skills: hand strength, hand-eye coordination, precision, refined movements, bilateral coordination.[1]

Babies tear paper. Hand them a children's book with paper pages and—rip! Within seconds, that colorfully illustrated book is destroyed. However, instead of becoming angry your baby tore the book, provide books with thick cardboard pages at this young age. Ripping paper is a typical developmental phase, where your baby is once again learning cause and effect.

Your baby's hands are impressive structures filled with small muscles and bones that eventually work together to develop incredible precision. The remarkable coordination your baby's hands will one day demonstrate is in the current trial-and-error development stage. Take comfort in recognizing the progress that has already occurred. At birth, your baby's hands were fisted, but your child can now move their fingers individually. For example, they can hold the paper with one hand and use their fingers on the other one to rip paper. Each hand is doing different motions to accomplish the activity. Your baby's development has advanced when each hand does different actions to achieve a task.

Tearing paper is one way babies strengthen those muscles and learn the precision necessary to accomplish the task. Instead of offering a book with paper pages, try wrapping some of your baby's toys in gift wrap or even butcher paper, then allow your child to tear into those items to their heart's content.

Offering a better alternative is less stressful than saying no frequently. For example, fill a container with a few wrapped items and sit on the floor alongside your child as they unwrap them. You can also act excited as they discover what appears. Always look for ways to make learning fun.

Ways to Encourage Your Baby's Development:

- Fill a container with scrap paper or odd bits of wrapping paper. Allow your baby to tear those but always supervise for safety.
- Provide a few books with thick cardboard pages your baby can handle. They're exploring books at this age. Hold off on buying books with paper pages until they're older.

Things to Remember:

I'll wrap a few of your toys and allow you to unwrap them.
I'll put away books you may tear up. When you're older, I'll bring them back out.

Chapter 102

Up and Down

It is common for babies to fall when they are learning to roll, crawl, walk, or stand. This is a normal and unavoidable part of development![1]

Independent mobility—rolling, crawling, or walking—comes with the risk of injury. For example, if your baby rolls off the changing table, they fall hard and fast to the floor. Other serious injuries can happen if they crawl down the steps or walk off the porch. While you expect falls to occur, do everything within your power to minimize how badly your baby can hurt themselves when they do. For example, never leave your baby on the changing table. Pad sharp edges and install barriers.

When your baby falls, remain calm as you hurry over and check them out. While this response is easier said than done, your child will look to you to see whether to be upset or scared. If you panic, your baby may feel unsafe. Modify your body language and voice level to help them calm down.

Babies eventually learn to fall without injury, and you can help develop that skill. Our bodies have automatic movements to prevent injury, such as extending our hands. Your child is learning those skills at this age. Allow your crawler to crawl onto a big pillow or couch cushions on the floor. When they tumble—and they will—the chances are slim they'll get hurt because they're close to the floor. Keep those cushions away from sharp edges, stairs, or other items you don't want your baby to hit if they fall.

Ways to Encourage Your Baby's Development:

- Place a couch cushion in the middle of the floor for them to crawl up and down. You can also use big pillows. The skills they learn by crawling up and down from these lower heights will eventually assist them when they begin climbing playground equipment.
- They can crawl up and down over you or another family member. Add in grunts and groans they may mimic. Daddies love this game, and it is good for both of them.

Things to Remember:

I'll clear out a space on the floor for you to crawl on pillows.
I can guide you up and down as you get used to this activity. Doing this will increase your confidence.

Chapter 103

Crawling Under

A potential link between laughter and language development suggests we've thus far underestimated babies' sense of humour.[1]

As your child becomes increasingly mobile—crawling all over the house—sooner or later, they'll end up underneath a piece of furniture. You may step back into the room and find them sitting quietly under the dining room table. *Are they hiding from me?* you wonder. Maybe they're playing hide-and-seek.

A baby of this age thinks that if they can't see you, you can't see them. They're still learning the cognitive concept of object permanence. You may think they should realize that if you see their legs, you see them. But they haven't learned that yet.

Hide-and-seek is an advanced version of peekaboo. Babies can't yet understand all the rules of hide-and-seek, but they're learning to hide and hope you find them. You may also enjoy hiding and encouraging your child to find you. These types of games, while silly and innocent, are beautiful forms of communication.

Have you discovered that your baby communicates quite a lot without using words? For example, they may have different cries for when they're wet versus hungry. They laugh at funny faces, and they may wave when you do. These are vital forms of early communication and socialization. So, play peekaboo, hide-and-seek, or catch-me-if-you-can.

They won't understand what it means to tag someone or how to be It for a while. But at this age, who cares? Giggles and laughter are the goal, because these forms of communication have immeasurable positive effects on your baby's social and language development.

Ways to Encourage Your Baby's Development:

- When your baby sits quietly under the furniture, act as if you don't see them. Say, "Where's (baby's name)? I don't see you!" Make a show of looking for them under the sofa cushions or other silly places, such as in a basket. When you stoop down and find them, say, "There you are!"
- Laughter is good medicine, and laughing with those you love is the best form of social engagement. Minimize competition for your baby's attention by turning off your phone, tablets, and televisions.

Things to Remember:

Some things that make you laugh are

____.

I'll find ways to laugh with you a few times each day.

Chapter 104

Pulling Mommy Over

There is no specific time and place to pinpoint the origin of tug of war. The contest of pulling a rope originates from ancient ceremonies and rituals, which are found all over the world.[1]

A fun way to help your baby gain strength in sitting is to play a modified version of tug-of-war. No, this activity won't teach your baby to fight or become aggressive. Instead, it engages your baby's natural instinct to make themselves laugh. Who doesn't want to hear a baby laugh?

Some kids need help to develop stronger core muscles, especially the abdominal muscles. This game has been a winner with almost every child I've tried it with. Even if your baby doesn't need more strength or better sitting balance, the game fosters social engagement and communication. Shared laughter is communication.

For this game, sit on the floor facing your baby. Place a few pillows behind your child to prevent a hard fall in case they lose their balance. Next, place a baby blanket or burp cloth between the two of you that both of you will pull. Make sure your baby can easily grasp the fabric you choose. If the baby pulls on it, you plop forward and do something funny, such as make a silly sound or a loud groan. Your baby may want to do this repeatedly.

You can also gently pull on your baby, not to pull them onto their face, but to give them the idea to pull back. Do your face-plant act to make them laugh when they pull. Those moans, groans, grunts, and funny faces are ones your baby may try to imitate. Great! These sounds are pre-word vocalizations that help babies eventually form words.

Ways to Encourage Your Baby's Development:

- If you don't enjoy playing this game with your baby, have another family member play it, such as daddy or an older sibling. Moms don't have to do everything to ensure everything gets done. Consider delegating.
- Your baby may enjoy falling backward on the pillows. If so, you can add funny sound effects when they land, such as "Boom!" or "Kaboom!" Warning: Lots of giggles may occur.

Things to Remember:

I love to hear your laugh.
I'll take a few minutes once a day to play this game with you or ask someone else to do it.

Chapter 105

Shake It, Baby!

A study published in the Proceedings of the National Academy of Sciences found that a series of play sessions with music improved nine-month-old babies' brain processing of both music and new speech sounds. According to the authors, the results indicated that experiencing a rhythmic pattern in music can also improve the ability to detect and make predictions about rhythmic patterns in speech.[1]

Babies often love music, and as they become mobile, they usually begin to move and bounce when they hear their favorite tune. While dancing comes later, your baby may bop and weave already. These are excellent skills your little one is developing. To ensure they're responding to music and not merely imitating the movements of cartoon characters, turn off electronic screens, such as televisions, tablets, and phones. See if they react to music without it being paired to a cartoon or video.

Sing familiar nursery rhymes, especially those with finger plays, including "The Wheels on the Bus" or "Baby Shark." In your country or community, there may be others. Sing or play the ones you like. You want your baby to learn your language. If you're one of the numerous multilingual families, include music from all the languages that make up your unique household.

As you sing or listen along with your baby, bob your head or sway your body so they learn to mimic you. You can also clap your hands or pat your leg to the beat. The more your baby attunes their ear to musical rhythms, the better their understanding of the rhythms of language will be.

Again, use music only. Many in today's culture overuse visual entertainment, such as watching cartoons or billed-as-educational videos, thinking these are the best ways to teach children. They are not. The children's games and songs that have survived the centuries continue to be the choice of therapists when it comes to helping your baby meet developmental milestones.

Ways to Encourage Your Baby's Development:

- Play music in the background during the day. Turn off background sounds—such as televisions, tablets, and phones—that interrupt your child's attention and interfere with deep listening.
- Learn and sing traditional nursery rhymes. Learn and do finger plays with your baby.

Things to Remember:

The first time you moved your body while listening to music was on

________________________.

Music enhances brain development, and the classical styles should be included. I'll add some classical music to the playlist.

Chapter 106

Clean Out the Basket

Silence is golden. Unless you have kids.
Then silence is just suspicious.[1]

If your baby is on the move, either rolling or crawling, you may have discovered the truth of the above quote. For example, perhaps your baby has crawled down the hall into their bedroom, and you no longer hear them. *Are they okay?* you wonder.

You hurry down the hall to ensure they're alive, only to find they're quietly pulling every toy out of the basket. There they sit, happy as a lark, surrounded by a mountain of toys and stuffed animals. Your first thought, hopefully, is relief that they're safe. Your second one is likely *Why are you making a mess?*

A quick reframing may help. Your child doesn't see the pile of toys as a mess. You see it that way. They see a mountain of exciting objects they've figured out how to get to by themselves. Recognize that they're doing what is typical for their age and praise their discovery skills.

Now that they can pull things out of containers, they can help you. For example, when you fold clothes, sit them beside your piled-high laundry basket. Allow them to pull out the towels or socks. Then reach your hand out and say, "Give it to me." They may or may not obey.

However, now is the time to take these newfound skills and weave them into ways your baby can contribute to the daily work of family life.

Instead of getting angry at the mess, make it work for you. Incorporate their new skills into helping with daily household tasks. Praise them for helping you.

Ways to Encourage Your Baby's Development:

- Fill baskets or plastic containers with everyday household objects, such as dishrags, potholders, wooden spoons, plastic measuring cups, clean brushes, sunglasses, caps, etc. If your baby is mouthing a lot, don't allow them to handle items they may break or that have small parts, such as sunglasses.
- Teaching your baby to give something to you on request is vital for their safety. Unfortunately, your child will pick up hazardous items. Therefore, they need to learn to hand an item over when told to do so. Also, when requesting they give you something, don't say, "Can you give me that?" or "Will you give it to me?" They may shake their head no. Use a directive instead, such as "Give it."

Things to Remember:

I'll let you pull clothes out of the laundry basket.
To build your vocabulary, I'll tell you the name of each everyday object as you pull it out of the container.

Chapter 107

All Done!

Around six to eight months old is a great time to start teaching your baby how to sign.[1]

Many parents think that if their baby learns some simple sign language, also known as baby signs, doing so will interfere with their child's talking. But that isn't true. Yes, every parent wants their baby to use words to communicate. For example, moms always want to hear mama, and daddies like to hear dada. Those are heartwarming words that build emotional bonds between parent and child.

As your baby gets older and more selective about what they do or don't want, you want them to tell you. Doing so will make everyone less frustrated—baby, you, and other family members. In early intervention, teaching baby signs is always recommended over continuing to wait for your baby to use words. For example, learning the sign for milk teaches your baby to ask for milk rather than handing you the cup and whining. Building this connection between an action and an outcome (what they want) is the beginning stage of learning to communicate specific wants and needs.

Many apps are available if you want to try teaching your child some baby signs. You don't need to teach letters, phrases, and sentences. You only need to introduce some words, such as *milk, mama, dada, drink, eat*, and *all done*. While apps may teach the sign for *more*, the speech pathologists I've worked alongside discourage using this general sign, as it can lead to more frustration for both you and the baby. For example, maybe your baby wants more milk and signs *more*. However, you don't know if they want more milk or more of something else. If they signed *milk*, you'd know.

As you use the signs, simultaneously say the word. Using the sign and word together helps your baby eventually say the word. And most children learn that saying the word is easier and faster than signing it. It never hurts to seek an assessment if you have concerns about your baby's communication skills.

WAYS TO ENCOURAGE YOUR BABY'S DEVELOPMENT:

- When you think your baby wants a drink, simultaneously sign *drink* and say it. Make sure they see you. Then hand over the cup. Please don't withhold the beverage if they don't make the sign. Doing so will increase frustration and diminish learning. Use this technique with all the signs you try.
- Begin with one or two signs. What sign should you teach? Ask yourself what specific thing your child could sign that would decrease frustration the most. For example, do you want your baby to be able to specify whether they want to eat or drink?

THINGS TO REMEMBER:

I want to teach you how to sign the words *eat* and *drink*.
Make the sign quickly, but don't expect your baby to imitate. Eventually, you may notice them attempting to make the signs with their hands. Praise those efforts!

Chapter 108

Baby Wants Milk

Breastmilk or formula is an important part of your child's diet until his first birthday. But from six months, milk alone can't provide everything he needs. In particular, he needs to eat some solid foods that contain iron, to make sure he's getting enough.[1]

Babies around six months of age are usually ready for pureed foods. However, if your child doesn't yet have steady head control or sitting balance, they aren't prepared. Your baby needs enough strength in the neck and torso to eat solid foods. Talk with your child's doctor if you have questions about your baby's readiness for solids.

Some babies love to suck on their mother's breast or the bottle. By the middle of your baby's first year, they should take supplemental nutrition via pureed foods. They'll still receive most of their nutrition via the breast or bottle for a while. However, some babies gravitate toward sucking on the nipple more for comfort than for sustenance.

Some careful observation may be in order. Babies need comfort, and sucking on a breast or bottle provides that. However, exclusively drinking formula or breastmilk doesn't provide adequate nutrients for them. If this applies to your baby, talk with their doctor.

Begin by offering one pureed food per week to see if your baby will eat it. Sometimes they will initially refuse or push food out of their mouths because it's new. However, their desire for pureed food usually improves with a bit of patience and time. Remain calm and avoid stress. Remember, babies pick up on your body language. Work to convey that all is well.

Always have your baby seated in a stable, upright position. Eating and swallowing food when you're reclined or lying down risks choking. The same goes for babies. Allow your baby to touch the food and don't insist on keeping them immaculately clean. The more they can handle and explore food, the more likely they'll continue to enjoy different tastes and textures.

Ways to Encourage Your Baby's Development:

- When you feed your baby, don't distract them with electronic screens (tablets, phones, or televisions). Instead, keep their focus on you.
- Have your baby join the family at the table for the family meals when you can. Family mealtimes connect us. Turn off other distractions and talk about pleasant subjects.

Things to Remember:

I'll make sure you're not drinking too much milk because then you won't be hungry for other foods.
Maybe I should offer a pacifier instead of a bottle when you need to suck for comfort.

Chapter 109

Hat Shopping

At 10 months, babies learn to grab and pull and take things off, like a sock, shoe, or hat.[1]

Many babies have grabbed and pulled off clothing long before ten months. Some learn later, and that's okay. If your little one needs more practice and will tolerate hats on their head, they may enjoy hat shopping.

Position them in front of a mirror and place a hat on their head. They may enjoy seeing it there. Describe some features of the hat, such as whether it's soft or firm, red or green, big or small. Allow them to pull it off and help as needed.

They may even try to put the hat back on their head. Let them try and help if they allow. It would be rare for them to get it on successfully at this age. You may recall that your baby is in the phase of taking things off, out, and apart. Later, they'll put something on, in, and together.

You can also do this fun game with other easy-to-put-on clothing items. Try shoes or sunglasses. Name the object and describe some of its characteristics. Talk to your baby about how cute they are and how the color complements their hair. Have fun!

Hat Shopping

If your baby hates hats or panics when something is placed on their head, put a hat on your head. Look in the mirror together. Have them pull the hat off your head. Maybe seeing you're okay with the hat on your head will alleviate their fears. Many children struggle to tolerate a hat, so it may be a while before they accept one. Continue to try. If you make the process fun, they may work through their fears faster.

Ways to Encourage Your Baby's Development:

- Offer a few hat choices for them to try on and take off. Seeing themselves in the mirror makes the experience more enjoyable. You can also snap a few photos and view those. Looking into the mirror, however, is the better choice.
- Print out a few photos of your baby wearing hats. Bring the pictures out occasionally and let your child see themselves in the photos. Talk about the characteristics of the hat, especially the color and style, such as ball cap or cowboy hat.

Things to Remember:

I'll find a spare hat or cap to use for this game.
When it comes to wearing hats, you ____________________them.

Chapter 110

Not Enough Hands

Sometimes the most important things you do each day are never even on your list.[1]

If you're like most moms, on many days you feel you don't have enough hands to complete everything on your to-do list. Even though moms are gifted at multitasking, juggling all the feeding, changing diapers and clothes, house duties, and their paid job takes it to another level.

While your baby isn't yet able to keep up with an adult's responsibilities, they're learning to use their hands to accomplish more than they could a few months ago. For example, now they pick up rattles and move them between their hands. They may also be able to pick up and hold two small objects simultaneously, such as a rattle and a teething biscuit.

You can add some more fun and challenge by laying out three of their favorite small toys. It could be a rattle, a teething ring, and a small block. When they have something in each hand, hand them the third one and see if they figure out whether they can hold all three or only two. Simple challenges like this aren't designed to create frustration.

Instead, they offer your baby a new problem-solving opportunity. Figuring things out is how all humans build brain power.

After your baby has eaten and is content, try playing this game in the high chair while you finish putting away food and cleaning up. Games like this one are better choices than turning on the television or watching a video on a tablet or phone. Better play choices equal better developmental outcomes.

Ways to Encourage Your Baby's Development:

- Offer your baby three small objects. These could be small toys or everyday items. See if they can hold all three or if they lay one down to pick up another. Either way, they're learning motor and cognitive skills they can't learn by watching a show.
- Label the items for them. "Here's your rattle, teething ring, and a blue block. Can you hold all of them?" The more words they hear, the more they learn.

Things to Remember:

The first time you held three items at the same time was on

_____________________________.

I'm amazed by how long you'll work on a task before getting frustrated.

Chapter 111

Put It In

By 9 to 10 months of age, your child can drop his toys into a large container with control.[1]

Previously, your baby was dumping and pulling items out of containers. They may have already dumped out all the blocks, cereal containers, and sock drawers, along with scattering the dog's chew toys across the floor. They've mastered taking things out!

Now you long for them to put objects back into the container from which they came, right? *Put your toys in the box, put those dirty clothes back into the hamper, put your food into your mouth and stop feeding it to the dog*—you may have had thoughts like these for weeks.

Your child is now at the age to learn the skill of putting things in. Putting stuff into the basket isn't as enjoyable as taking everything out, but that's a topic for another day. Help your baby learn to put items into containers by encouraging them to copy you. Drop the block into the box and say, "You do it." Maybe you can add the request, "Help Mommy." Young children often love to help. While their help may create more work for you, encourage them to help anyway.

Expect their attempts to be imperfect. Tap into their curiosity to help. Perfecting the task will take a considerable amount of time, but you're teaching that you expect them to assist with simple everyday tasks.

During the activity, repeatedly say the word *in* as the toys or blocks drop into the container. Saying a word again and again cements it into your baby's memory faster than hearing the word every once in a while. For example, if you say "in" each time you drop a piece of cereal into the bowl, they may hear the word fifty times, right? While you'll tire of it, recall those silly songs on your baby's favorite shows. You've listened to them until you're sick of them. But you memorized them, didn't you? Repeatedly hearing something sticks in your memory, and it will do the same for your baby.

WAYS TO ENCOURAGE YOUR BABY'S DEVELOPMENT:

- Dropping blocks or balls into a container repeatedly is a beneficial game to play a few times each day. If you don't have time, delegate this activity to another family member, like daddy.
- Non-interlocking blocks offer better opportunities for your baby to refine their grasp and hand dexterity. Wooden ones with colorful letters, numbers, or pictures will be useful to teach a variety of concepts over the coming years.

THINGS TO REMEMBER:

I'll buy some wooden blocks.

The first time you learned to put an item into a container was on

____________________________.

Chapter 112

Mommy Said No!

Babies understand that "no" means "no" around 9 months if used firmly and consistently. But consistent use is not the same as overuse. Save "no" for dangerous behaviors such as touching the stove or going near electrical sockets.[1]

A curious, on-the-move baby can get into danger quickly. For example, you glance down at your phone to check on something, and before you know it, the lamp falls off the end table because your tot has crawled over and found the electrical cord. Then with a quick jerk, the lamp crashes onto the floor. Or your child rapidly crawls into the kitchen, and before you catch up, they're munching on the pet food, and the water bowl is upended.

When it comes to the word *no*, most mothers go from hoping they'll never have to use it to overusing it. If you have an active child, you may overuse too.

For your child's safety, they need to learn the meaning of the word *no*. At this age, when a child is told no, they briefly stop before continuing. They may turn and look, giggle, or smile before returning to their plan. They're not intentionally disobeying or misbehaving because they don't yet understand the dangers of what they're doing. But your child needs to learn to stop when given a firm no. That's the reason you want to avoid overusing it.

Use redirection when you can. For example, if your baby is pulling items out of the drawer, offer another toy and transition them away from the activity you prefer they don't do. Say, "Let's play with your blocks!" or "I see you want to pull things out. Let's get the clothes out of the basket." Using these transitional phrases and redirection methods takes practice. However, eventually it will create fewer frustrations and meltdowns. Use no when you must, such as when your child bangs their toy on the glass-top coffee table.

Ways to Encourage Your Baby's Development:

- Use a firm tone when you say no. Firm, deeper voice tones gain more attention.
- Practice using transitional phrases and redirection to a safer choice when your child is getting into something they shouldn't. Save your no for dangerous situations.

Things to Remember:

The first time you stopped when I told you no was on

______________________________.

While I wish you'd stay out of some things, I admire your perseverance.

Chapter 113

What's That Sound?

By 6 months, your babies should be turning their head or eyes toward the source of sound.[1]

By now, your baby should be turning to look for who or what made a particular sound. For example, if daddy comes home and turns on the television, your child not only hears it but also turns to look. Likewise, if you call your child from across the room, they should turn and look. While they won't do this 100 percent of the time, they should do it most of the time.

Earlier, I addressed how background television noise competes with you for your baby's attention. For example, suppose your child isn't consistently turning to look for a sound or a voice. In that case, first try turning off the television and keeping it off. While both of you may miss the sound, detoxing from excess noise may be necessary.

A fun way to help your child look for and identify sounds is to use some of their favorite toys that make noise, such as musical toys or books with push-button sounds. Make a sound with one of those toys while your baby isn't looking. When they turn, say, "What's that sound?" Show it to them and repeat the sound. For example, say, "It's your rattle!"

What's That Sound?

You can use everyday objects like keys, shakers, bells, or crinkly paper. Try to use naturally occurring sounds more than electronically generated ones. For example, use a real bell instead of a bell sound on your phone. The tones are different, and naturally occurring tones generate more interest. You can clap your hands under a blanket, whistle while hiding behind your hands, click your tongue, or blow raspberries. All of those sounds your baby can also make or at least attempt.

Ways to Encourage Your Baby's Development:

- Make various sounds using toys, objects, or yourself. Encourage your baby's interest in finding where the sound came from or what the sound was. For example, if you clap your hands under the blanket, when your baby pulls the blanket off, say, "I'm clapping my hands!"
- If your baby has a book with buttons that make sounds, such as a cow mooing or a chicken clucking, imitate those sounds and see if your baby can moo or cluck. Refrain from asking, "Can you moo like a cow?" Instead say, "Moo like a cow."

Things to Remember:

I'll buy some baby-safe musical instruments, such as bells, tambourines, and drums.
I'll encourage my baby to click their tongue and smack their lips to make sounds.

Chapter 114

Fist Bump

By 8–12 months, most babies may even play patty-cake or give you a "high five."[1]

Different cultures have different gestures for greeting, agreeing, or offering praise. For example, today many offer a fist bump. Not long ago, the high-five hand slap was a typical gesture. In the future, some other gesture may arise. Since your baby mimics actions, you may have introduced him to the fist bump or a similar gesture.

It's an important milestone for your baby to acknowledge and greet the presence of others in some way. Maybe your younger brother comes home, and fist-bumps everyone. Your baby should be encouraged to join in. Or you give a fist bump when someone does something good or achieves a new skill. Do the same with your baby. If they finish their food, offer a fist bump, high five, or something similar. I've evaluated many babies who attend church regularly. When the praise music starts, they raise their hands in praise. These gestures indicate that your baby is learning to join others and do what they're doing. Great!

An old saying goes, "Be careful what you say and do 'cause little eyes are watching you." That's as true today as it was long ago. Your baby is watching you closer than you realize. They may seem disinterested or preoccupied, but they're hearing and imitating. So, monitor what they hear and see. Many mothers cringe when their child blurts out an inappropriate word or makes an offensive hand gesture.

Create an environment where your child hears positive words and learns uplifting messages and gestures. Demeaning verbal or gestural communication does nothing to build a more loving world. Set the example in your home, and when you do, we'll all give you a fist bump of praise.

Ways to Encourage Your Baby's Development:

- When your baby completes a task successfully, such as feeding themselves, give them a fist bump or some other gesture of praise. Encourage them to seek recognition from you. Doing so is an indicator of advancing social skills.
- If you allow your child to view television shows, ensure they're appropriate for your child's age. Adult themes and language don't contribute to creating a kinder, gentler world for our children.

Things to Remember:

The first time you did a fist bump or high five was on

______________________________.

I'll ensure that you aren't exposed to adult-themed shows or violent video games.

Chapter 115

Mommy Kiss It

We've always thought that smooching our kids' injuries only "helped," thanks to the placebo effect. But new science shows that kisses from mom may actually have real healing power![1]

A recent study revealed that the saliva released by a parent when kissing a child's injury might boost healing. While no one is advocating licking the wound or spitting into a cut, it does make one wonder whether a mom's saliva has real power to heal.

A mother automatically kisses her baby's bumps, cuts, and bruises. She also kisses her child to ease hurt feelings, wounded pride, and disappointments. Kissing your little one creates an emotional connection and shows you care. When your baby feels loved, their body releases oxytocin, a naturally occurring hormone that makes them feel better. And a mom always wants to ease the suffering of her child. Doing so comes naturally.

Since your baby is moving around, exploring, and getting into everything, bumps and bruises happen, sometimes hourly. So, you'll have many opportunities "to kiss it and make it better." Kiss those knots on their head and their pinched fingers, then cuddle them.

To teach your baby to care for others, ask them to kiss your hand if you smash your finger. If you're sad, request a cuddle and a kiss on the cheek. You're teaching them to be aware of the feelings of others and helping them learn to show concern.

Every mother wants a kinder, gentler world for her child. Home is where that better world begins. While you can do little about what happens in the homes of others, you can create a home where caring for others is demonstrated and expected.

Ways to Encourage Your Baby's Development:

- Kiss your baby's hurts—physical wounds and emotional bruises. Show you care.
- If your baby slams their teddy bear down or drops it on its head, pick it up and kiss it. Doing so is a simple way to teach your baby that their actions can harm.

Things to Remember:

I want my baby to care for the needs of others.
I'll teach you how to kiss and comfort me when I'm sad.

Chapter 116

Baby Faces

Researchers say infants develop the ability to imitate during the second half of their first year of life, mostly between 6 and 8 months of age.[1]

Most babies love staring at their mom's face. Human faces are one of a baby's preferred objects of interest. Looking into your eyes, swatting at your nose, and maybe imitating sticking out their tongue are everyday activities for babies. If your child loves these activities, you probably do them together frequently.

However, if your baby isn't doing any of them and seems to look anywhere but at you, please talk to your pediatrician. While no one wants to hear about possible autism, some early signs of this condition show up during this age; however, difficulty making eye contact or engaging with others doesn't mean your child has autism.

Some of the characteristics of autism are challenges with social skills, repetitive behaviors, and communication delays. A few early red flags are poor eye contact and a lack of imitating facial expressions. While autism isn't usually diagnosed in babies, early identification of red flags may allow you and your child to receive help. If you have questions, get help. Don't "wait and see."

I've evaluated many children with poor social skills who prefer watching cartoons or videos on tablets or smartphones to interacting with real people. Moms want to keep their babies happy and often allow their children to enjoy what they love. However, children who don't engage with others can get lost "in their own world." For many babies, their preferred world is one of cartoon characters. However, that isn't the world in which we live and must interact. In these cases, doing what they love is unsuitable for their development. While challenging, mothers should always do what's best for their children, even when the baby prefers something else.

Ways to Encourage Your Baby's Development:

- Discontinue using the television, tablet, or phone to keep your baby happy. Begin a new routine by reducing the usage by one-half per day. For example, if your child watches a thirty-minute show, reduce the time to fifteen minutes. Continue for a few days, then wean again. Strive for zero.
- Fill the time during which your baby used to watch shows by playing with your child. The goal is to make the real world more interesting than the virtual world.

Things to Remember:

I'll wean my baby off watching so much electronic entertainment.
I'll talk to your doctor if you don't make good eye contact with me.

Chapter 117

Are You Sad?

When you label emotions of people in your environment (especially when strong emotions are witnessed), or those your baby expresses, you give words to feelings and reassure her that feelings of all kinds are valued.[1]

When a new mother becomes emotional, it may be difficult for her to label those feelings. Is she crying because she's sad or overwhelmed? Did she laugh because something was funny or because she didn't want to cry?

Learning to label our emotions is an important skill. For example, when we recognize that we're sad, it helps us seek and discover the reason. Doing so can teach us to better understand why we feel as we do and what we may do to feel better.

Teaching your baby in the early years to label their emotions will help them throughout life. For example, when they cry, say, "I see you're sad. Did you hurt yourself?" Looking at picture books with faces that express different emotions—such as sadness, happiness, or fear—will help your child learn to identify those expressions on others. Giving them the words to describe the feelings on those faces helps them label them.

Then one day when their friend cries, they'll realize their friend is sad. We comfort those who are unhappy, and you've taught your child how to do so. If you're scared, they'll see that and one day ask you, "Mommy, are you afraid?" Begin today to teach your baby the words that describe how they and others feel.

Ways to Encourage Your Baby's Development:

- In front of a mirror, mimic certain facial expressions, such as sad or happy. For example, tell your baby, "Mommy is sad" or "Mommy is happy." See if your baby can imitate some of those faces.
- Use a book that contains pictures of faces expressing different emotions. Point to one and say, "He looks sad" or "He seems to be afraid." Get a book with cardboard pages so your baby can explore it without tearing it apart.

Things to Remember:

The first time you imitated a sad face was on

______________________________.

I'll label what you feel so you can learn those words.

Chapter 118

Over My Leg

There are two main types of baby crawling: belly crawling and hands and knees crawling. Unlike belly crawling, which relies on coordination of the same-side leg and arm when fully mastered, hands and knees crawling requires coordination of oppositive-side limbs.[1]

Maybe it's just the families I've interviewed over the years, but many mothers seem to believe that skipping the crawling phase and going straight to walking is somehow the better route of development. Is this a case of mothers wishing their children to have superior abilities? Maybe so.

I also wanted my children to excel; however, skipping important milestones is like running a marathon without learning how to complete a 5k race. Multiple levels of achievement contribute to meeting the overall goal. For example, crawling on hands and knees is a crucial building block for walking. Some children skip crawling on hands and knees, and they're "doing fine." Those instances, however, shouldn't lead you to assume all similar cases will have the same result. Babies crawl on their hands and knees for a reason.

Just as your baby learns to do more with their hands, such as picking up small items or dropping a ball, they must also learn to move their opposing arm and leg in opposite ways. Crawling on all fours and walking are such skills. When crawling on hands and knees and walking, one arm and the opposite leg, such as the right arm and left leg, move in concert. These are advanced movement patterns you want your baby to achieve.

So, try not to skip hands-and-knees crawling. While your baby may not achieve this critical milestone despite your efforts, do your best to ensure they have adequate learning opportunities.

Ways to Encourage Your Baby's Development:

- If your baby struggles to get on their hands and knees, sit on the floor and place them over your leg so they're on their hands and knees. You'll have to help them stay, but your leg will help support them.
- While they're over your leg, look at books or place a mirror on the floor to interest them. Don't expect them to stay there for more than a minute or two. Come back to this activity multiple times during the day, but don't make it a battle.

Things to Remember:

The first time you balanced on your hands and knees by yourself was on _______________.

I'll offer you more time to play on the floor or in a playpen.

Chapter 119

Let's Swing

The assumption is that because they were often in motion in the uterus, they'll love a similar motion after being born, but a swing is not a natural motion, and not all babies will like it.[1]

Some babies love their baby swings, and others don't. No matter how fancy yours is, and some are elaborate, many babies don't tolerate the swinging motion. Each of us has a vestibular system that gives information about movement. For example, this system lets you know whether you're going forward, sideways, or upside down. Explaining the way it works would fill a book. But for this discussion, understand that your baby's vestibular system is developing.

You may love roller coasters now but didn't as a child. Or you may be like me and no longer love fast and twirly rides. Your baby currently loves certain toys and activities, but their preferences may change over time. For example, they probably won't love mashed squash or green peas in kindergarten. Therefore, if your baby dislikes their swing now, please don't assume this dislike will continue.

Just because your baby tolerated motion in utero or when rocked doesn't mean they'll like a swing's linear motion. These motions are different. For example, some swings go forward and backward, and some go side to side. These aren't naturally occurring planes of motion. We don't move side to side like a pendulum on a clock on our own. Instead, even though we walk forward, we display a bit of body rotation.

If your baby dislikes swinging, try swinging them while you hold them. Feeling your touch may ease the anxiety. Start with small ranges of motion but don't force them to do anything that causes panic. Over time, they'll become more comfortable swinging.

Ways to Encourage Your Baby's Development:

- Introduce your baby to a swing by standing in front of it where they can see you. Swinging in small arcs as you face them may ease fears.
- Always have your baby in a swing that offers adequate support and security. Always buckle your child in and ensure they have sufficient head control for this activity.

Things to Remember:

I'd like to buy you a baby swing for outdoor play.
Holding you on my lap while swinging on a porch swing is a good idea.

Chapter 120

Baby Standers

When your child is placed in a device, that device hinders your baby from learning how his body moves without being contained in a device. When your baby is placed on the ground instead, your baby can explore how he rolls, scoots along the floor, and transitions between different positions.[1]

When your baby begins scooting around the house, you may think you need a baby stander, stationary play station, or exersaucer. While keeping your baby safe as you attend to other duties is a good idea, placing them in a stationary position for longer than a half hour isn't wise.

Your baby is learning how to move, and moving is what they do. Using their newfound mobility to explore and learn about the world is your baby's daily work. Unfortunately, sitting in an immobile play station stops exploratory movement.

When your child is in a stander—where they can sit and move their body back and forth without falling—they aren't learning that those same motions will result in falls when not contained within this equipment. If they stand on their tiptoes, they're using the wrong movement pattern. Standing on tiptoes isn't how we stand. We stand flat-footed.

Developmental experts, like pediatric physical therapists, always discourage the use of baby standers. While some recommend getting rid of them, others will allow them for short periods. But none of them will encourage their use. Why? There's no developmental upside to their use. No stander or play station will help your child learn to stand or walk. Your child has to learn those skills without the support of a piece of equipment. They have to learn to balance and how to fall, and standers prevent learning those skills.

Ways to Encourage Your Baby's Development:

- If you use stationary play stations, limit them to no more than thirty minutes twice a day. Use them only when you can't supervise your child, such as when you prepare a meal.
- Playpens are better choices for keeping your active baby safe. In them, they can crawl and pull to standing without you worrying about them getting into unsafe areas.

Things to Remember:

A safe play area or playpen is better than a stationary play station or baby stander.

Using a stander while you watch a TV show won't help you meet your developmental milestones.

Section Four

Ten to Twelve Months

Chapter 121

Don't Want

Facial expressions, gestures, and body language all play a role in expressing ourselves, interpreting what others are saying, and how well others understand what we say.[1]

Every mother wants to converse with her baby. She wants to know how they feel or what they want to eat. You may already dream of hearing your child read a story or tell you about their day. Those days will come. But today figuring out whether no means no is the order of the day.

By this age, your baby may start shaking their head to indicate they don't want something. While they figure out how this communication works, expect them to make many mistakes.

For example, you offer them their favorite blueberry pancake, and they shake their head no. They may even push it away. Since they adore this breakfast item, you're surprised. "Are you sure?" you ask. Again, they shake their head. They're trying out their new powers to get their wants and needs met; however, they rarely know what they want at such a young age.

A sense of humor helps you maintain your sanity during this

phase. As your child learns to gesture what they want, expect crying and fussing because they'll change their mind frequently.

Communication with babies becomes more challenging the more they attempt it. Taking care of a baby was more manageable when you knew they needed either feeding, changing, or sleep. Now, they want this and not that. Or at least that's what they think they want. So, as they begin expressing themselves, be patient.

Ways to Encourage Your Baby's Development:

- Model shaking your head when you say the word no. For example, when they toss their bottle on the kitchen floor, shake your head and say, "No, don't throw. Give it to Mommy."
- If they shake their head or push food away, remove the food. Let them begin to understand the consequences of saying no.

Things to Remember:

You're so cute when you tell me no.
The first time you shook your head no was on

________________________________.

Chapter 122

Waving Hello

Between 8 and 12 months, many babies start to wave "hello" and "goodbye."[1]

Your baby may have imitated the waving motion for a few months. For example, when daddy left to go to work, you and baby waved bye-bye. The sitter and your child waved when you left to pick up groceries. Hopefully, there were only a few tears. By this age, most babies learn the concept that people come and go. They've paid attention to what others do in these circumstances and are learning the social skill of greeting.

When you come home, you expect those already there to greet you. Maybe your husband kisses you or looks up and says hi. Your child may go over and reach for you or wave hello.

Babies don't see the hello wave as often during daily life as they observe the bye-bye wave. Many families don't regularly wave hello. Instead, they greet in other ways, such as hugs, fist bumps, or saying hey. What you want your baby to learn is to welcome others in whatever way your family does it.

Many of today's families have a home filled with electronic distractions for babies, such as constant television noise, voice-activated home controls, or electronic tablets. You may have noticed that your child is so focused on other objects they barely acknowledge when you come and go. Why? You may be less interesting than their video. One way to change that scenario is to turn off electronic devices.

We all want to be greeted and missed. Show your baby you missed them by waving hello upon your return. Please hug and kiss them to show you're happy to be back. The more your child learns these standard greetings by seeing them expressed in their home, the more likely they'll retain and use them.

WAYS TO ENCOURAGE YOUR BABY'S DEVELOPMENT:

- Model waving hello when others visit or when you meet someone while running errands.
- Wave hello to your child's favorite stuffed animal and say, "Hello, Mr. Bear!" Encourage your baby to greet the animal too.

THINGS TO REMEMBER:

The first time you waved hello was on

____.

We'll practice greeting pets and people when they enter the house.

Chapter 123

Holding the Spoon

Babies can start to use a spoon by themselves at around 10 to 12 months old.[1]

While it may be a while before they can scoop and feed themselves, your baby is likely reaching for the spoon every time it gets near their mouth. Once your baby learns to feed themselves finger foods, they seek more control and may grab at the spoon. Knowing they'll make a huge mess, you don't give it to them. But is that best for your baby's development?

There are many differences of opinion on this topic based on cultural preferences and family traditions. Some families I've worked with over the years don't allow their babies to get messy during eating. Others allow their tots to make huge messes and seem to care less about the cleanup required.

However, if your baby doesn't hold or practice using a spoon, they won't learn to do so anytime soon. I suggest giving your child a spoon to hold while you use another one to feed them, which should decrease their keen interest in taking a spoon from you. Allow them to try to scoop by placing a small amount of food on their high-chair tray or in another container.

Holding the Spoon

If your child struggles to hold the spoon and make a scooping motion, let them practice scooping water into a container during bath time or digging in the sandbox. The dig and scoop motions are the same whether they're scooping sand into a bucket or pudding into their mouth. To build their vocabulary, continue repeating the word *in* each time they get the spoon's contents into the container.

Ways to Encourage Your Baby's Development:

- Experiment with various spoons—lightweight plastic baby spoons and heavier metal spoons. Some babies do better with a heavier spoon.
- If your child insists on trying to use a spoon to feed themselves but can't get the food into their mouth, place your hand over theirs to guide the contents into their mouth.

Things to Remember:

You began holding your own spoon on

______________________________.

I'll allow you to hold a spoon while you're being fed.

Chapter 124

Pulling to Standing

Usually around 7–12 months babies will start pulling themselves up to stand.[1]

Suppose your child has been crawling on hands and knees. In that case, chances are they'll soon be grabbing onto you or the furniture and pulling themselves to a standing position. Some children who haven't crawled on their hands and knees may do this also, but usually they're unable to get onto their knees and balance.

Pulling to standing is one of those milestones often delayed when a child doesn't crawl or has played a lot in a baby stander or jumper. Those babies haven't developed the ability to get onto their knees and pull themselves up. Their bodies are too weak because they lack the hours of practice spent getting in and out of the sitting position and crawling around.

Also, some babies prefer to be held in the standing position and have minimal ability to transition in and out of this position without help. For your child to be safe when standing, they have to eventually learn how to get up and down from standing without falling. There's no way to learn these motions other than doing them.

If your child has avoided crawling and prefers to scoot on their backside or wiggle on their tummy, you may have to guide them onto their hands and knees. Help them kneel while holding on to you or a sturdy stool. Let them figure out how to get down without your help. Falling from this height is less dangerous than from a standing position.

WAYS TO ENCOURAGE YOUR BABY'S DEVELOPMENT:

- Place some firm cushions or pillows on the floor. Encourage your baby to climb on and off so they can learn how to balance on their knees.
- Encourage your baby to push toys while on their knees. For example, pushing heavy toys or boxes will strengthen their legs and core.

THINGS TO REMEMBER:

The first day you pulled yourself into a standing position was on

________________________.

I'll remove some of the sofa cushions so you can easily pull yourself up to standing.

Chapter 125

Pincer Grasp

The pincer grasp is the ability to hold something between the thumb and first finger. This skill usually develops around 9 to 10 months old.[1]

Your baby's hands are remarkably complex structures. They've progressed from the newborn phase of reflexively grasping your finger to picking up a small piece of food using only the thumb and first finger. The pincer grasp gives your child a remarkable level of skill and fine motor coordination. While your tot's school days seem a long way away, the pincer grasp is the foundation for their ability to firmly grip a pencil.

One of the easiest ways to help your baby master a pincer grip is to allow them to practice picking up small bites of food and feeding themselves. Spread out each bite-sized piece of food so your little one is less inclined to scoop up a bunch in their hand. For example, many children don't want to eat one piece of cereal at a time. Instead, they prefer to shovel in a couple with each mouthful. Spreading out the bits discourages this behavior.

If your child still tries to rake and shovel, offer only one piece at a time. Continue to offer practice during meals. You can also provide toys that require your baby to poke one finger into a hole or to push a button using the pointer finger. If your baby prefers to use their thumb or another finger, help them press the button with their pointer finger.

Ways to Encourage Your Baby's Development:

- Many of today's children have weak hands because they prefer playing on electronic screens, such as tablets and phones. Screens require a light touch, but flipping switches and pushing buttons in the physical world require more strength.
- Pop-up toys with various switches, such as buttons to push, slides to move, and knobs to twist offer opportunities for your child to develop good grip and hand strength.

Things to Remember:

The first time you used a pincer grasp to pick up your food was on

____________________.

I'll buy you a pop-up switch toy to improve your finger dexterity and hand strength.

Chapter 126

Where Did It Go?

Perform a simple test. Show a child a popular toy. Hide it under a blanket as he watches. Observe the child's reaction. If the child attempts to lift the blanket to grab hold of the toy, it is safe to assume that he understands object permanence, at least partially.[1]

In earlier chapters, I discussed variations on the timeless game of peekaboo. Of course, by this point, your baby may have advanced in their abilities and now tries to cover their face to play. Or they're hiding under furniture and waiting to see if you find them. Another variation on finding hidden objects is to cover a favorite toy and see if your baby uncovers it.

Make sure they see you cover it and use a small towel or blanket they can grasp and lift. Always make the activity fun and exciting. When you cover the toy, say, "Where'd it go?" See what your baby does. Do they wait for you to uncover it, or do they try to do that themselves?

When the toy is found, say, "There it is!" and act excited. Exaggerate your reaction because babies love drama. Even if you're a quiet person, add a bit of enthusiasm a few times a day. Increase the suspense by looking under other objects first, saying, "Is it under the couch?" or "Is it under the chair?" Many babies love for you peek under their bib or shirt and say, "Is it under here?" Giggles often result.

Ways to Encourage Your Baby's Development:

- Use a small toy your child enjoys and cover it with a blanket. You can also use everyday items your child finds interesting, such as keys or the remote control. Avoid using the phone.
- If your child is struggling with this activity, use a toy that lights up or a flashlight—seeing the light may increase your child's curiosity and motivation.

Things to Remember:

I'll encourage your grandparents or other family members to play this game with you.
I'll hide your pacifier or bottle under the blanket to see if you can uncover it.

Chapter 127

Give It to Me

You could take your kids to a restaurant or cut out the middleman and just spill a drink, throw crayons under the table, and light $40 on fire.[1]

Once your baby learns to toss things, expect food to hit the floor. The bottle or sippy cup, rattles, bibs, and anything else those little hands can snatch and throw will fly. At first, it was cute, right? But now your back aches from repeatedly picking up stuff from the floor. And if you've taken your baby out to eat, did you pick up all those French fries, or did you sneak out hoping no one noticed your child made the mess?

The cause-and-effect game where your baby tosses something and you give it back has gotten old. So, what can you do? Maybe it's time to teach a new game called "Give It to Me."

Your baby is learning gestures, such as pushing items away or turning their head, indicating refusal or disinterest. They may reach for you when they want you to pick them up. I suggest you try the gesture of holding out your hand and saying, "Give it to me" or "Give it to Mommy." When they finish their bottle and sling it, pick it up, hand it back, then hold out your hand and state, "Give it to me." Help them place the item in your hand and praise them by saying, "Thank you!" or "Great job!"

It'll be a while before they routinely hand an item to you before tossing it. Still, they'll eventually learn the meaning of the gesture and command. You can also practice with toys or items of clothing. When they pick up the blue block, extend your hand and say, "Give it to Mommy." Always praise the effort and don't persist to the point your child is frustrated. A disappointed child is rarely compliant.

Ways to Encourage Your Baby's Development:

- Encourage other family members to teach "Give it to me." The more your baby hears this helpful command, the faster they'll learn it.
- When you tell your child no, add a preferred action. For example, you can say, "No, don't throw it. Please give it to me."

Things to Remember:

The first time you gave an item to me upon request was on

______________________________.

To make the after-meal cleanup easier, I'll place a plastic tablecloth or shower curtain liner underneath your chair to catch food and liquids.

Chapter 128

A Climber

Climbing is part of the natural progression ever since your baby learned how to pull themselves up. It's no surprise that once they can defy gravity and stand without holding on, they want to do it more and more.[1]

Once babies learn how to crawl, climbing often begins. They may crawl up onto pillows on the floor or up the steps. As they begin to pull up to a standing position, they may hike their leg to try to get up onto the sofa. Some babies are more adventurous than others, and you may prefer your child not to climb. But climbing builds strength, confidence, and coordination.

If your tot is a climber, create a safe environment for them to explore. My youngest child was a climber, and it was impossible to stop him from climbing. Maybe that will be your experience too. However, you can embrace their need to push the limits by creating safe climbing areas. Putting big pillows on the floor, such as removable sofa cushions, is one option. Indoor climbing equipment may be within your budget, and many climbers love those.

Children who climb are often strong and coordinated. They excel on the playground and move confidently. However, they can also be risk-takers and lack good judgment regarding safety. Be vigilant and watch your child closely. Avoid nagging or yelling at them to stop climbing. Instead, create safe climbing opportunities. You can also try to transition your climber to another activity by telling them what activity is next, such as, "It's time to take a bath." Don't ask, "Do you want to take a bath?" The answer will often be no. Please don't allow them to tell you no when you won't accept no as an answer.

As your baby learns to say no, learn how to give directions rather than ask for their permission. If no isn't the answer you want, then don't ask the question. Instead, make a declarative statement of what's next on the schedule.

Ways to Encourage Your Baby's Development:

- Make sure your baby can't climb out of the crib—lower the mattress to its lowest level.
- Temporarily remove coffee tables or other furniture that could topple onto your child. Create safe climbing areas because no matter how much you try to stop the climbing, your child will persist for a while.

Things to Remember:

I'll block you from climbing stairs or over barriers to get into the bathroom or laundry areas.
I'll store all dangerous liquids, such as cleaning supplies or laundry detergent, where you can't reach them.

Chapter 129

Pushing the Furniture

Parenthood is a journey except it's just traveling from room to room putting away the same toys all day long.[1]

When your baby begins to crawl on hands and knees or pull to the standing position, they may start pushing furniture. Some babies move objects while they walk on their knees. For example, they may push large trucks or boxes across the room or pull up on your kitchen chair and try to slide it across the floor. Moving items is another form of exploration your baby enjoys.

This activity is still part of the cause-and-effect phase of play. For example, when they push on the chair, what happens? They learn the chair can move, and they will fall. And unfortunately, they'll fall many times before gaining the balance necessary to stay upright. Besides climbing and exploring, pushing objects is another way your baby explores the environment to discover what happens when they do certain things.

My youngest son was a climber and a pusher. He was so insistent on pushing the kitchen chairs around the room that I eventually put them in the garage. No chairs equal no danger. I could no longer stand the worry he'd get hurt, and I couldn't keep redirecting him without losing my patience. So, the chairs went bye-bye. We also had to remove the glass doors from our entertainment center because he repeatedly pushed and banged on the panes. After a year, the phase had passed, and the doors returned.

If your baby is pushing your furniture around or turning over the coffee table, preserve your sanity. Eliminate the dangers by removing furniture for a while. The peace of mind is worth the small sacrifice in how your house looks during this phase of your child's development. At least, I thought so.

Ways to Encourage Your Baby's Development:

- Offer a thirteen-gallon plastic storage box with a secure lid. Fill it with blankets to give it weight. Encourage your baby to push it around.
- Fill a laundry basket or box with tightly capped two-liter soda bottles. Allow your baby to push it around.

Things to Remember:

I'll offer other items for my baby to push around the house.
The pushing-the-furniture phase will pass.

Chapter 130

Making Mommy Laugh

Researchers at the University of Portsmouth found that from the age of seven or eight months children intentionally use their faces, bodies and voices to make adults laugh or smile.[1]

A sure sign of advancing social and emotional development is your baby initiating activities to make you laugh. Maybe they're covering their face with a blanket and then uncovering it, seeking your attention and laughter. Or they may spontaneously make funny faces they've learned, such as sticking out their tongue or blowing raspberries. Playing games with others is an important milestone.

Many of today's children spend more time watching cartoons than playing games with others. Patty-cake, peekaboo, and even "I'm going to get you" build relationships. Children need stable, loving relationships with family. While giggling at a cartoon is fine, your child isn't developing or enriching social relationships with others while watching the show.

Pediatricians recommend no screen time for babies. While few families meet this goal or attempt to, one thing is sure: today's kids are bored and lonely. Lack of relationships with friends and family is the root of the problem. And it starts early. Is your baby watching TV shows more than playing with others?

Your child needs playmates. Check local churches for mom's day out programs or try the childcare at your fitness center. You can also connect with neighbors or friends who have young children and organize some weekly playdates. If nothing is available, start your own playgroup.

Ways to Encourage Your Baby's Development:

- When your baby initiates a game, do your best to play along, even if you only participate for a minute or two.
- Educational shows or videos don't teach your child how to relate better with others. In fact, they do the opposite by allowing your baby to disengage from others and be in their own world.

Things to Remember:

The first time you made me laugh with your antics was on

____________________________.

Use a mirror to practice funny faces and make each other laugh.

Chapter 131

Watch Me

Not only does screen time not deliver benefits for babies and young toddlers, it can actually negatively affect language development, reading skills and short-term memory, according to the AAP[American Academy of Pediatrics]. It can also disrupt a child's sleep and capacity to pay attention.[1]

Screens are everywhere. Most babies have watched something on a smartphone or tablet. Babies seem drawn to these devices like a bee going for nectar. What's a mother to do?

Most moms allow their babies to watch shows and videos. For example, while standing in the checkout line or waiting at the doctor's office, the baby wants the phone. If mom doesn't hand it over, the crying begins.

The science is quite convincing that screens are harming young children. Today's kids have shorter attention spans and more language delays than previous generations. Many demonstrate poorer imaginative and pretend-play skills. The apparent reason is today's babies sit and watch moving objects on screens more than they move themselves and engage in other types of play.

If you want your baby to watch you and learn how to get along with others, work toward setting up a home where those activities are preferred. For example, turn off televisions and put away tablets and phones. Let your baby engage more with the natural world and less with a digital imitation of one. Richer language, greater creativity, and better engagement with others should result. Still not convinced? Try it for a week and see what happens.

WAYS TO ENCOURAGE YOUR BABY'S DEVELOPMENT:

- If your baby seems distracted or isn't turning when their name is spoken, say, "Watch me!" This phrase may draw their attention. Touching your child on the shoulder may also help them focus on you as you speak.
- Felt boards, cloth books, and other non-electronic toys are better choices than anything battery-operated.

THINGS TO REMEMBER:

I'll stay off my phone as much as possible when I'm with my baby.
I'll purchase some non-electronic toys for you to play with.

Chapter 132

Comforting Others

As infants grow older and more mobile, they begin to comfort distressed others in more complex ways, such as by giving objects that they think will be comforting.[1]

Your baby may pat your back or hand you a toy if they see you're upset. If another child cries, they may look at the baby to see what's happening. Most children by this age no longer cry when another child cries, but they are curious. They're showing they're in the early stages of noticing the needs of others. While they remain focused on their own needs most of the time, they're realizing others also have needs.

Many moms automatically fake cry to see what their child does. This is an effective way to model sadness to help teach your baby to check on others and offer comfort. For example, you could make a pouty expression and say, "Mommy's sad." Labeling the emotion enhances your child's understanding of feelings and how to identify them.

Children often automatically offer to share toys or bring other items to show as they seek to engage with others. When your child brings you a toy, they seek to interact with you, so maximize those moments. Unfortunately, many of today's children lack good engagement skills and an understanding of how to comfort and care for others. Some role-playing with baby dolls or stuffed animals can help. Say something like, "Is your baby crying? Pat them on the back, so they feel better."

These phrases and actions seem simple, and they are. But simple doesn't mean unimportant. All the fancy, expensive electronics in the world can't replace these time-honored interactions between one person and another. But unfortunately, such engagement is missing for many of today's children. Instead, youngsters prefer to interact with characters on a screen. As a result, they're unaware of and lack sensitivity to others' needs. You can change that in your home by choosing different play activities and the back-and-forth interactions you have with your child.

Ways to Encourage Your Baby's Development:

- Pretend to cry and ask your baby to pat you on the back or hug and kiss you. Teach them how to comfort and care.
- Playing with baby dolls or stuffed animals offers opportunities to kiss that hurt foot or comfort the teddy bear. Both boys and girls love to show concern and give attention to the needs of others.

Things to Remember:

The first time you patted my back to comfort me was on

____________________________.

When you pat too firmly, I'll say, "Use soft hands."

Chapter 133

Roll It Back

For little kids, playing is everything—fun, yes, but also vital for their growth.[1]

For months, your baby has played with toys, such as rattles, push-button toys, or mirrors. By now, they should be playing with you. Peekaboo is one of the first baby games children play. Most babies love it. Your child may also have played chase as you crawled after them down the hall. They may have handed you a toy, such as a book for you to read to them. By the end of their first year, they should be rolling a ball back and forth.

I've evaluated many children who've never played the simple game of sitting on the floor and rolling a ball back and forth to another person. Instead, today's children are often left to play alone or plopped in front of the television to be entertained. When I discover these situations, my heart is always sad.

While most moms buy balls for their babies, few parents play ball with their young children. I'm not suggesting you spend the whole morning playing ball instead of tending to the other vital duties on your list. However, I encourage you to take a few minutes each day to sit and roll a ball back and forth with your child. Maybe do it after dinner instead of watching a show or engaging in roughhouse play, which makes it challenging to get your child to sleep. Rolling a ball back and forth is an excellent game as the baby winds down for rest.

To add a little more to the activity, when you push the ball forward, say, "My turn." And, when your child rolls it to you, say, "Your turn." Teaching these phrases helps them learn about taking turns. Learning to take turns and share is essential to enjoying play with others.

Ways to Encourage Your Baby's Development:

- Sit on the floor facing your child. Be close enough to touch each other's feet. Slowly roll the ball forward to your child and encourage them to roll it back.
- If they lose focus and try to get up and move around, encourage them to "sit down and try again." Regular patient practice will reap benefits. Do a session or two each day.

Things to Remember:

We'll roll the ball back and forth, one session each day.
The first day you rolled the ball back to me was on

________________________________.

Chapter 134

Turn It

By 11 months, babies learn to turn things. They can turn a ball on their toy mobile, a steering wheel on a toy car, or the faucet in the tub. They can turn a page in a book. And they can turn a basket upside down, put it on their head, and make you laugh.[1]

Can your baby turn things? For example, are they turning the steering wheel on the toy car or turning a key on the dashboard? Many pop-up toys have a knob to turn, like turning the key in a car. While turning it every time they try will take a while, they should be figuring out how to do it by now.

Many children miss this skill because they have no toys with knobs to turn. Instead, all they have are push-button toys. By this age, your child needs to learn more challenging switches, such as sideways slides, up-and-down slides, and knobs.

As your child learns to flip and turn switches, they strengthen their hands plus improve their problem-solving cognitive abilities. Figuring things out builds brain power. Sitting and watching someone else do it on television or on a video doesn't. Your child must figure it out physically to master the skill.

Take inventory of the toys your child plays with. Do any of them have various types of switches or knobs to turn? Your baby should also be able to turn objects over and look at the underside. If they struggle, you can help by doing hand over hand as they turn the knob. Let them feel the motion.

Ways to Encourage Your Baby's Development:

- Ensure your baby has toys with switches and knobs. Making a busy board for your child is a great DIY project.
- Help your baby turn a knob or an item over by holding your hand over theirs. Allow them to feel the movement as it happens.

Things to Remember:

The first time you turned a knob was on

______________________________.

I'll help you turn knobs or wheels during playtime.

Chapter 135

Flip the Switch

People often say that practice makes perfect. Research certainly supports this, especially in children.[1]

When my child began climbing up the back of the couch, he always wanted to turn the light switch on and off. Over and over, over and over. Light on, light off. It was funny and cute for a while, but I soon became annoyed.

Your baby is learning a lot when they reach high, stand on tiptoes, point a finger, and flip the light switch. Keeping their body balanced while doing this complex movement with their hand is a significant accomplishment—one we adults take for granted. When your baby discovers the light switch, they find another fantastic cause-and-effect toy. Flip the switch up and the lights come on. Flip the switch the other way, and the room becomes dark. So much fun!

Yes, they've mastered a considerable motor accomplishment. But having the lights flicker on and off can be nerve-racking. You might think once they flip the switch a few times, they've learned the skill. However, children love doing things repeatedly. Have you noticed they love you to read the same book over and over? Or they have a strong preference on which blanket they want for sleeping? Children crave predictable routines and structure. And their daily play involves lots of repeated actions. This is how they learn.

Adults also repeat actions. For example, did you take lessons in music or sports? If so, you recall practicing the fundamentals again and again. Mastering those basic movements increased your skill. Your baby is no different.

Ways to Encourage Your Baby's Development:

- Provide toys that include various types of switches, not just buttons to push.
- Old-fashioned rotary or push-button phones offer beneficial play opportunities for your baby to learn how to poke a finger in a hole and turn the wheel or push a button. Look for old phones in a yard sale or second-hand store.

Things to Remember:

I'll find some toys with switches and rotary dials for you.
The stronger your hands, the better you'll write, use scissors, and trace when you're older.

Chapter 136

Simple Puzzles

Babies start to work with simple, one-piece puzzles around 6–8 months.[1]

Simple, one-piece puzzles are best for your baby at this age. Large pieces with big knobs your child can easily grasp are ideal. Look for ones with circles, squares, and triangles. Other shapes are too complicated for babies under one year and are more appropriate during the toddler years.

Many conscientious moms teach their babies colors and shapes using flash cards. A better choice is physical puzzles, such as the one described above. Don't be fooled into believing that when your baby matches shapes on an electronic screen, they're completing a puzzle. They aren't. They haven't mastered puzzles until they can physically place a puzzle piece in the correct place.

To explain all the body systems your baby uses to see, pick up, rotate, and place a puzzle piece into the proper position would fill another book. By comparison, touching a digital button on the screen to make another digital image pop magically into the correct spot is elementary when compared to the difficulty of mastering the completion of a real puzzle.

Simple Puzzles

While your baby doesn't yet need to learn shapes and colors, you can still tell them the shape and color of each puzzle piece. However, please refrain from academic memorization drills using flash cards. For most children at this age, play activities using the hands and bodies are preferable to visual memorization. Play is supposed to be fun, and memorization drills aren't usually fun.

Ways to Encourage Your Baby's Development:

- Offer one- or two-piece puzzles for your baby to play with. Select ones with large knobs and durable construction.
- Your baby will bang and slam puzzle pieces during this period of learning. Again, purchase ones with large knobs and sturdy construction.

Things to Remember:

I'll make a list of the toys that would be most suitable for your first birthday.
Most babies master placing the circle long before other shapes.

Chapter 137

Sippy Cups

Richard Belanger devised the unique spill-proof spout mechanism that characterizes all modern sippy cups. He licensed his patent to Playtex in 1981.[1]

For many centuries, mothers raised their babies without sippy cups. What did they use? Regular cups, and there were lots of spills. Somehow, I doubt those moms allowed their babies to carry a cup around the house. But they also didn't have to drive everywhere and balance a job outside the home. At least, most didn't.

Sippy cups are a mainstay today. But they aren't without some naysayers. For example, some speech and language pathologists prefer skipping sippy cups and transitioning to straws or an open cup with assistance. And some mothers have no intention of weaning their babies off the bottle or breast by one year and see no point in giving their child a sippy cup.

But if you consider using them, most babies can begin trying them by six months. Expect to try various styles before finding the one your baby likes. You may decide, as many mothers do, to use the sippy cup for all drinks except milk. Some children won't drink milk from a cup;

they always prefer a breast or bottle. Whatever cup you choose, always clean the spout or straw well.

Many mothers also allow their babies to drink from the sippy cup during the day and let them move around with the cup. That's your choice. However, drinking while moving around isn't recommended.

Sippy cups are a luxury item, so don't fret if your child refuses. Children born in the United States before 1981 learned to drink from a cup without them. And millions of children throughout the world have no access to these conveniences and learn to drink from a cup. Your baby can too. The only reason to use a sippy cup is to decrease spills and minimize the workload of the caretaker. Your child has no inherent need to master one.

Ways to Encourage Your Baby's Development:

- Offer water in the sippy cup during meals. Allow your child to handle the cup to get comfortable with it.
- Straw cups are popular. However, your child doesn't need to tip those back to drink. When your child learns to drink from an open cup, they have to learn the tipping motion. So, you'll have to deal with spills, either now or later.

Things to Remember:

When it comes to sippy cups, you _________them.
The first time you drank from a sippy cup was on

____________________________.

Chapter 138

Baby Talk

As babies continue to develop, their babbling begins to sound more and more like conversation. This is sometimes referred to as jargon, and this babble has a rhythm and tone which sounds a lot like adult speech.[1]

Most babies are babbling by the end of the first year. Some talk a lot; others are quiet. There is wide variation in this; however, your baby should be babbling and making sounds. For more vocal children, many have advanced from babbling to jargon. For example, you may hear them talking to the dog, which sounds like a conversation. But you don't understand a single word.

Some describe their baby's jargon as sounding like they're speaking another language. Speech like that is typical. As your baby talks more, act like you know what they're saying. For example, "Yes, I see that you spilled your drink. Do you want more?"

The more you converse with your child, the more they should talk to you. With time and practice, their babbling should begin to approximate words—*nana* for *banana* or *baba* for *bottle*. Perfect pronunciation takes years. Don't fret about whether the words are pronounced accurately. Instead, work on helping your baby communicate using gestures and babbling.

Always discuss specific concerns with your doctor. If you have early intervention services in your area, seek an assessment from a professional. In the meantime, talk to your baby. Say the words you believe they're attempting so they hear them pronounced correctly. For example, when they point at the car and say, "ca," you say, "Yes, that's a car."

Ways to Encourage Your Baby's Development:

- Babies who watch a lot of television or videos can display delays in speech development. Babies learn to talk so they can engage with others. If your baby prefers engaging with a TV show, they have less desire to talk to you.
- If your baby babbles something, reply with "Really? Tell me more." Using this prompt may get more back-and-forth talking going. It doesn't matter if you understand a word said. Act interested.

Things to Remember:

Some of your words are

____.

Most babies begin babbling with common consonants *b*, *m*, *p*, and *d*.

Chapter 139

Bringing Toys

Most children develop sharing abilities around 3.5–4 years old, not at 1–2 years as many expect.[1]

Sharing is hard for everyone, so it must be taught. Babies at this age aren't yet capable of understanding the concept of sharing. While some of your child's actions, such as trying to put some of their French fries into your mouth, appear to you as sharing, experts say it isn't. Trying to feed you or hand you a toy are ways to gain your attention. Give positive attention to your baby when they give you something.

You may want to say, "Thank you" when your tot feeds you some cereal. In addition, you could sign thank you. Babies pick up these easy-to-make signs quickly. For example, if they hand you a crayon, say, "I love blue. Would you like to color with me?" Use simple phrases that convey doing things together.

During these months, expect your baby to take back what they offer. They're learning what you'll do when they give or take away. For example, if they snatch a toy or other item away from someone—and most children do at some point—calmly react and say, "Let's share and give them a crayon. Then we can all color together."

Also, if your baby takes back what they handed you, you could say nothing or you could take the opportunity to build some language skills and say, "I guess you changed your mind. Maybe I'll use this yellow crayon while you keep the blue one."

Ways to Encourage Your Baby's Development:

- Manners can be taught early. Babies learn simple signs quickly, such as please and thank you. It's never too early to begin.
- If your child snatches a toy away, understand they're too young to be mean. They want everything for themselves, which is typical behavior at this age. Therefore, we begin teaching manners at this age.

Things to Remember:

I love it when you try to feed me.
I'll teach you the signs for please and thank you.

Chapter 140

Going for a Cruise

Babies generally start cruising within weeks of learning to pull to stand, usually between 10–12 months.[1]

Not long after your baby begins pulling to stand, they take a step or two sideways while holding on to the sofa or coffee table. For example, they may see the television remote control and step over to grab it. As they practice, expect them to lean too far and fall. Eventually, they'll learn to sidestep rapidly up and down the couch. When they do, they're going for a cruise.

Cruising furniture allows your baby to strengthen the muscles on the sides of their legs—the ones they use to sidestep. They'll need those muscles to walk and run safely. Encourage your baby to cruise by placing a favorite toy just out of reach. When they stand at the sofa, they'll see it and figure out how to reach it. Always ensure they can't hit their head on anything hard or sharp if they fall.

Allow your baby to practice this skill while barefoot as much as possible. Tons of sensory information is conveyed from your child's feet to their brain, so letting their foot feel the floor is ideal. However, nonskid socks and shoes with soft soles are fine when the weather is cold.

Going for a Cruise

Babies who've spent too much time in jumpers, stationary play stations, or baby walkers don't learn to cruise as early as unrestrained babies. That type of equipment prevents your baby's legs from learning how to step sideways or how to balance as they shift their weight from one leg to another. If you need to keep your baby contained for safety, a playpen is a better choice because it allows your baby to cruise.

Ways to Encourage Your Baby's Development:

- Place exciting toys along the sofa so your baby can cruise sideways to get them.
- Bare feet are ideal as your baby learns to stand and walk. Make sure their socks and shoes have nonskid soles.

Things to Remember:

I'll encourage you to cruise while I sit on the sofa.
Your pack-n-play is also a place where you could pull up and cruise.

Chapter 141

Calming Down by Myself

It's usually best to encourage self-soothing behaviors before separation anxiety kicks in full force, around 8 to 9 months. It can be hard for your little one to learn to soothe themselves back to sleep when they're already worried about being separated from their favorite adults.[1]

When your baby can soothe themselves back to sleep, you may believe you've reached the end of this going-without-sleep phase. Self-soothing, though, is a hit-and-miss accomplishment with children. They've learned to calm themselves when they put their pacifier in their mouth or go back to sleep after a few minutes of babbling. Celebrate this achievement. However, as with many aspects of raising babies, sickness, teething pains, or the emergence of new fears create setbacks. Therefore, retraining is an ongoing activity.

You should allow your baby to calm themselves. Don't run and attend to every whimper. You may assure your child from the doorway without touching them or rub their back without picking them up. If your baby wants to be touched or held, it'll be hard for them to learn to go back to sleep without your presence. Not picking up a fussing child is difficult and may seem cruel. However, you shouldn't ignore a panicked child. Don't run to check on a child who whimpers or fusses a little but isn't waking up the entire house—just you. Teaching your baby to self-soothe takes time but is worth the effort.

Ways to Encourage Your Baby's Development:

- Try using a nightlight in your child's room. A bit of light may calm their fears.
- Work toward calming them with softly spoken words and refrain from touching or picking them up.

Things to Remember:

Keep their sleeping area free of items that could smother them.
I'll move your crib into my room instead of putting you in the bed with me.

Chapter 142

Come Here

Parenting hack: There are no hacks. Everything is hard. These kids don't listen. This is your life now. Godspeed.[1]

Once your baby is on the move—crawling or walking—they'll get away from you. You'll find yourself repeatedly yelling, "Come here!" Then, for maybe the first time in your baby's life, you'll call them by their full name. Every child knows that when mom uses their full name, she's angry.

Your child has become independent, so they must learn to follow your command to "come here." These types of phrases are considered safety words. Others are *no*, *stop*, and *give it to me*. You may have already panicked when your baby picked up a choking hazard and put it in their mouth. Or executed Olympic-worthy feats when you caught your baby before they crawled off the bed.

You've entered a new mothering phase filled with days of fun and exhaustion. You've been sleep-deprived, but now you'll also be physically exhausted from keeping up with your baby. For example, you're locking down cabinets, stepping over baby gates, and constantly cleaning the floors of choking hazards.

To teach your child to come, use the hand gesture meaning "come here." We all know it because we instinctively bend our fingers toward our palm to indicate "come back to me." Calling your child's name is an excellent first step. Do they respond to their name? They should be turning or looking up by around four to six months when they hear it. Discuss this situation with your child's doctor if your baby isn't consistently responding when you call.

Ways to Encourage Your Baby's Development:

- When your baby sees you, say "come here" as you gesture. Use a firm and slightly deeper tone of voice. When they move to you, praise them with, "Great job! You came over when I called you."
- Background noises, such as nonstop television sounds, can interfere with your child's attention. For example, if they prefer the show over you, you may need to stop competing with the television and turn it off.

Things to Remember:

The first time you came when I called you was on

________________________________.

Your biggest accomplishment this week is

______________________________________.

Chapter 143

Turning On the TV

It turns out that there is a perfectly reasonable scientific explanation for why kids love the remote control. The University of Saskatchewan wrote that toys (or non-toys, as it were) like these are multifaceted for children.[1]

Numerous studies have demonstrated that when babies are offered toys versus everyday objects, they usually choose the object. For example, if you handed your child a toy remote and a real one, my money says they'll pick the real one. And, if you placed a ball and a set of car keys on the table, they'd prefer the keys.

The remote control is fascinating to your baby. First, it has so many buttons to push or chew on (beware of this choking hazard), plus it often has lights. They may have discovered it turns on the television and can even find their favorite show. Or they know to hand it to you so you'll turn on the cartoons. What's not to love? Second, they see you use it often and copy what they observe.

While it's lovely when your baby learns how to use the remote, it's also maddening. No matter where you place it, they seem to know where the remote is and work to retrieve it. My suggestion is to wave as you say, "Bye-bye, remote," and put it out of reach and sight. When they fuss for it, say, "It's gone bye-bye." They're learning that phrase, which may help them understand why it's gone.

Ways to Encourage Your Baby's Development:

- Don't leave the remote controls where your baby can reach them. The buttons and batteries, if they become loose, are choking hazards. Instead, place them out of sight and reach.
- Teach your baby to say bye-bye to the remote when it's time for it to go away for a while. Consistent routines of putting it away when the show is over will help your child tolerate the transition.

Things to Remember:

I'll turn off the television when your show is over and not leave it on in the background.
I'll place electronics, such as game systems and movie or music players, out of reach and sight.

Chapter 144

Hold My Hand

When do babies start walking? In the United States today, the average age of independent walking is approximately 12 months.[1]

In the United States and worldwide, much variability exists regarding when most babies walk without help. The range continues to be as early as nine months and as late as eighteen months. These ranges have held true for decades regardless of baby equipment, culture, or financial resources. So, if your baby isn't yet walking, that's okay.

About three months before they take steps by themselves, your child may begin to walk when you hold their hands. Some children, however, won't walk when you hold their hands. Instead, they sit. I've seen many children do this. Often, the baby fears falling.

During this phase of development, some sensory issues may become noticeable, such as gravitational insecurity. We all have multiple sensory systems we use to balance and walk. However, in some babies, one or more of those systems isn't providing adequate feedback to your baby's brain. For example, maybe they don't feel their feet as well as they should, or they feel imbalanced when they can't hold on to something as sturdy as the sofa. There are many other possibilities too.

Continue to offer your hands to your child and encourage them to take steps. If they're hesitant, hold their hands in front of them instead of above their head. That may help. Once your child begins pulling themselves up to stand and cruise, give them time; if they don't get going, however, talk to your baby's doctor.

Ways to Encourage Your Baby's Development:

- Kneel in front of your child and hold their hands, then encourage them to walk toward you.
- Say, "Come here and give me a kiss," as you encourage them. Maybe getting to you will motivate them to try harder.

Things to Remember:

The first time you took steps while holding my hand was on

____________________________.

There is much variability in when children start walking. Each baby develops on their own timeline.

Chapter 145

Going to the Store

Be pre-emptive. Don't take a tired, hungry child anywhere.[1]

Take your child to the store or out to eat enough times, and eventually, your baby will act out or completely unravel. You'll feel other people's eyes of judgment on you, which happens to every mother sooner or later. Parenting is hard enough; criticism from others rarely helps. Have you been the target of unwelcome advice yet? If not, you will be.

As your baby gains greater awareness of people, they may suddenly be afraid of strangers and act out. Or they see all those exciting items on the shelves and want them. They don't understand why they can't get down and explore.

There are many ways to make taking your baby out into the community easier. My best advice is always take care of your baby's needs before or during the outing. Never, ever take a tired or hungry child anywhere. While some trips are unavoidable, you can usually schedule others around your baby's schedule. Your life will be easier if you can run those errands when your child is fed and rested. And always take snacks and a toy for your child to hold and enjoy.

Use the store as an opportunity to point out books or balls. Smile and engage with others and get your child used to how life functions outside the home. But, on the other hand, expect your child to be a bit overwhelmed with all the hustle and bustle and visual stimulation. An overwhelmed child often acts out, so make those trips quick and try to do them when your baby is rested and fed.

Ways to Encourage Your Baby's Development:

- On outings, take a toy or book for your baby. Don't rely on videos or games on your tablet or phone.
- Give your baby a snack while shopping or waiting at a restaurant. Keep them fed and happy to ensure a pleasant outing.

Things to Remember:

I'll put together a "trip bag" for outings.
I'll resist the urge to buy you a treat or toy every time we shop.

Chapter 146

Copying Words

Watch what you say and do because little eyes are watching you.[1]

Your baby may be imitating sounds or even first words by now. They may be babbling mama, dada, papa, and baba or talking up a storm in what sounds like a foreign language. You've probably learned their sounds and deciphered their vocalizations at this point. But don't be surprised if you're the only one who does. Even dads rarely understand baby talk as well as moms do.

What would your baby's first true word be if you could get your wish? Mama, right? Of course it is. Every mother, if honest, wants *mama* to be her baby's first word. Most moms also don't want one of their child's first words to be a curse word. Some mothers may not care, but I haven't met many of those. While it's wonderful that children learn by watching and copying, the older they get, the more they see and hear. Did they hear that ugly word on television or on a video game? Did they hear you say it when you slammed on the brakes driving to the doctor's office?

Babies pick up words by hearing them. What kinds of words do you want your baby to use? Do you want them to be a caring, kind child who encourages others and tells the truth? Or do you want them to be unkind and say words that hurt the feelings of others?

Children learn what they see and hear at home. You are your baby's first and most influential teacher. Embrace the role and begin modeling the behaviors you want your child to exhibit.

Ways to Encourage Your Baby's Development:

- If you say a curse word, apologize to your baby. Maybe offer a correction, such as "I meant to say, "Oh, no!" We all make mistakes, and you can teach your baby that you apologize and make it right when you do.
- Be vigilant about what words and behaviors your child sees on television shows, movies, and video games. The content is often inappropriate for young children.

Things to Remember:

The words you're saying now are

____.

I'll control the content you see on electronic screens, especially advertisements.

Chapter 147

Are You Listening?

A child's failure to consistently respond to one's name by their first birthday is often one of the most consistent early indicators of autism spectrum disorder and other developmental delays. This does NOT mean your child has autism—or any other condition. But it could.[1]

Every parent worries about an autism diagnosis. The condition is so prevalent that doctors routinely screen for it during office visits. Most everyone has met someone touched by this ever-expanding condition.

Not answering or responding to being called is a primary indicator of a possible autism diagnosis. I emphasize *possible* diagnosis. If you're concerned about your baby not responding when you call, don't panic; however, do a few checks as a precaution.

First, make sure they can hear. As discussed earlier in the book, stand behind them and shake your keys. Do they turn? Clap your hands loudly or drop a book on the floor. Did they acknowledge the sound by turning to look? If they did, they can hear.

Second, turn off all competing background sounds, such as televisions and music, and don't test while they're watching a show on a tablet or phone. They'll be mesmerized by the screen and tune you out. When all is quiet and calm, call them. Did they turn?

I've evaluated many children who didn't respond when called by name. Instead, they were glued to the screen and spent a lot of time doing that activity. Unless your child finds you more interesting than those shows, as I've stated before, you'll lose this competition for their attention. Stop competing with those shows if you want to improve their focus and interaction with you. Turn off the devices and keep them off.

WAYS TO ENCOURAGE YOUR BABY'S DEVELOPMENT:

- If your baby has allergies or multiple ear infections, request a hearing check from your pediatrician. For example, fluid in your baby's ears muffles sounds and may prevent them from hearing you call their name.
- Keep your house quiet so nothing is competing with your voice when you talk to your child. You want your voice to be the most interesting sound they hear.

THINGS TO REMEMBER:

I'll stop scrolling the internet and making myself afraid of possible diagnoses.

Many services are available to assist me if my child shows signs of autism. I'll talk to the doctor and seek help.

Chapter 148

Mama!

Taking care of someone else takes a lot of energy and giving up the lifestyle and your identity before you had children, while it may be everything you've ever wanted, is a hard transition.[1]

While you adore your baby calling you mama, on some days you wish they'd never learned the word. They cry mama every time they get hurt or feel hungry. They babble mama when they want a friend or when they're tired. Mama can fix it, so they call. You're the solution to all their problems. Your needs come second.

However, you do have needs, and maintaining your health, both physically and mentally, is not something to deny. A dry well has no water. So, when you feel empty and drained, you have nothing left of yourself to give. As a result, moms get burned out, and when they do, angry outbursts, crying jags, and depression may follow. You don't want that to happen.

By this age, if your baby is in a safe area and isn't hurt, it's okay to wait a bit when they fuss and cry. Maybe watch them from afar so you can monitor them, but they can't see you. Let them work longer to figure out that toy or allow time for them to find their pacifier to self-soothe.

Take three slow, deep breaths. While you wait, remind yourself that one of your jobs is to teach your baby some independence. If you always fix everything, that's what they'll learn. Ensure they're safe and give them time to solve their own problem. Their confidence will soar, and you can save your energy for when you do need to come to the rescue.

Ways to Encourage Your Baby's Development:

- If your baby isn't calling you mama, play peekaboo. When you appear, say, "Here's Mama!"
- Babies often call everyone mama for a while. While that may break your heart, don't take it personally. Your baby is practicing the word and will soon learn that you alone are their mama.

Things to Remember:

Some of the people you call mama are

__________________________________.

Whether you call me mama or not, you know I'm your mother.

Chapter 149

Directing Your Hand

By 12 months, your little one will turn pages (with some help from you), pat or start to point to objects on a page, and repeat your sounds.[1]

Reading books and looking at pictures in a book are ideal ways to help your child develop an extensive vocabulary. However, reading stories may not work for your wiggly child with a short attention span. Books containing pictures of faces, animals, objects, and vehicles are better choices. But for goodness' sake, make it enjoyable!

When you point to the sheep, say "baa baa" or say "woo woo" when you point to the firetruck. Add exaggeration and drama to your voice to increase your baby's interest. Even if you aren't a dramatic person, act like one during book time.

Help your baby point at the picture by placing your hand over theirs. They may grab your hand and make you point when they want you to say a word or make a sound. When they do this, celebrate! They're showing you what they want by taking control of your hand. Eventually, they'll point at things themselves. But for now, they use your pointer finger.

Directing Your Hand

They may also direct your hand to make you play peekaboo or get their cup. These actions are early forms of communication. To enhance their vocabulary, always label the item they point at—whether they use their hand or yours. Labeling objects at this age builds vocabulary.

Ways to Encourage Your Baby's Development:

- Point at pictures in a book and label them. Don't use a lot of other words. For example, say ball, cup, cookie, or dog. Avoid long phrases, such as "Oh my goodness, look at that cute dog" or "There's a red firetruck, and it's big and loud." Repeatedly saying single words is an excellent strategy at this age.
- If your baby directs your hand, say, "Show me." This will teach them to show what they want. Next, reciprocate and say, "You show me." Then take their hand, point, and label the picture.

Things to Remember:

You first directed my hand to what you wanted on

______________________________.

To increase your interest in books, I'll buy some with touch-and-feel pictures.

Chapter 150

Favorite Toys

By 9 months, your baby may have favorite toys and can interact with them by moving items from one hand to another or searching for a toy he sees you hide.[1]

Most babies at this age have a preferred item, whether it's a favorite blanket or a particular toy. When your baby was younger, they played with or explored whatever they picked up. They put it in their mouth, looked at it from different angles, banged it, and dropped it. But now, they have one or more objects they prefer, especially when sleepy or fussy.

By trial and error, you quickly figure out what those items are because you want to keep your baby happy. Make sure the items they enjoy are safe to put in their mouths and chew on because they will put them into their mouth. As their teeth come in, your baby chews and gnaws to relieve the discomfort. Always be safe.

Some babies have too many toys and become unfocused as they play. For example, they may pick up one toy and see another, drop the first one, then scramble over to the other. It's wise to limit your child's choices. The fewer available toys, the more they will explore each one. Helping your baby develop good attention and focus is an important goal. Also, avoid having multiple toys that do the same thing, such as light up when you push a button. Build variety in your toy selection.

Ways to Encourage Your Baby's Development:

- Babies need a toy or blanket to snuggle. Make sure no buttons, appliques, or decorations can become choking hazards if your baby bites or rips them.
- Encourage your baby to explore each toy more by limiting the choices at any given play session. Put some toys away and out of sight. Rotate your selection every week or so.

Things to Remember:

I'll buy you a stuffed animal or a soft blanket for snuggle time.
I'll put some toys away while you're sleeping.

Chapter 151

Standing Alone

Everyone talks about baby's first steps—but what about baby's first stand? It may not be a motor skill with quite as much celebration, but hey, it's still a pretty big deal![1]

Most babies begin to stand without support before the end of their first year. As with any of the milestones, each child develops at their own pace. Every mom eagerly awaits those first steps and has her camera ready. Walking is exciting, but your child won't walk until they can stand. And standing is difficult.

Many parents hold their baby in a standing position beginning in the early months. If you did this and your child seemed to stand and take a step or two—with your support, of course—you may have thought your baby would walk early. However, what you saw during those early months were typical reflexive movements. Reflexive movements aren't the same as purposeful motions your baby controls.

Standers, baby jumpers, and baby walkers seem to strengthen your child's legs to help them walk. However, I've not found this to be true. Many children struggle to learn how to stand because they practice the wrong motor patterns when they bounce and jump. The muscles your baby uses to stand on their own have various functions. For example, the ankle muscles are necessary to stand on tiptoes and flat-footed. For standing on tiptoes, the muscles move the ankle joint. To stand on flat feet, they maintain a steady ankle position.

For your baby to learn how to stand, those muscles must learn to hold position and balance. Your tot isn't learning how to stand and be still while bouncing around in a jumper or exersaucer. They'll master standing alone by practicing the skill without help. Until they can stand reasonably well, they aren't ready to walk.

Ways to Encourage Your Baby's Development:

- Encourage your baby to stand by the sofa or coffee table. Cruising and moving from one piece of furniture to another is how they learn to balance.
- Falling during this phase is expected. Remove or pad all sharp edges on furniture, hearths, or other household items.

Things to Remember:

I'll be patient. You'll stand and walk when you're ready.
The first day you stood without any support was on

______________________________.

Chapter 152

Showing Fear

Between 8–12 months of age—around the same time they understand the meaning of a fearful face—babies begin to produce fearful expressions and other fear-based behaviors, like clinging to a parent, making distressed sounds, or turning away.[1]

Each home is different. Some parents enjoy scaring their babies and even film the event. Social media is filled with parents making jokes about how scared their baby is. Other parents find no humor or entertainment value in intentionally making their children feel afraid.

Babies are seeing the world for the first time. Some of the most beautiful moments of parenting are discovering the world through your child's eyes, such as enjoying their excitement as they marvel at bubbles. Seeing them afraid shouldn't be fun. Fear is never fun for any of us.

Your baby may fear activities or circumstances they shouldn't be afraid of—for example, panicking when you wash their hair or screaming when you leave to go to the bathroom. Some of these are common for this development phase, such as stranger anxiety or fear that you aren't coming back. Other fears are often related to sensory dysregulation, such as panic when taking a bath or touching the sand.

We all have unwarranted fears, such as fears of roller coasters or the dark. Babies are the same. You can help them get used to some of those fears; others may require professional assistance. Mocking or belittling your baby's fears isn't recommended. Fear is a natural emotion, and it never disappears simply because someone says it should.

Ways to Encourage Your Baby's Development:

- Encourage your child to try and do new things, with your help if necessary. Activities may include touching bubbles or washing hair. Be patient. But if your child's fear doesn't seem to be a phase, talk to their doctor.
- Some babies are more sensitive to certain objects or situations than others. Maybe your child's sensitivity reveals a future talent. For example, many artists, musicians, and writers are more sensitive to the world than others are. As a result, your child may develop unique talents.

Things to Remember:

Things you fear or sensations you hate include

____.

Things I fear or sensations I hate include

____.

Chapter 153

Beware Blue Light

The screens of televisions, smartphones, tablets, computers, gaming systems, and certain e-readers all produce artificial blue light.[1]

Nature provides blue light from the sun. Science has shown the blue light from nature helps us sleep by regulating our sleep-wake cycle. The blue light emitted from electronics, however, is artificially generated and has been shown to interfere with that naturally occurring cycle. Just read the news; getting enough sleep is a problem for everyone, not only mothers.

Suppose you've found yourself too wired to sleep after scrolling social media or watching television. In that case, blue light exposure may be the culprit. Of course, viewing exciting content bears some blame. However, we already know modern-day humans sleep less than they did before the discovery of electricity. So, something is to be said for eliminating excess light from your room to get better rest.

The blue light emitted from screens interferes with the body's release of melatonin. Your body secretes melatonin to make you sleepy. If you don't have enough melatonin in your body, you won't sleep well. The same happens to your baby. The screens trick your baby's brain into thinking it isn't time to sleep.

Beware Blue Light

Your baby's eyes are also vulnerable to retinal damage from blue light. Many moms put sunglasses on their babies and coat them with sunscreen to prevent skin damage from harmful sun exposure. But many don't protect their children's eyes from blue light damage.

If sleep is an issue for your child, eliminating your baby's exposure to electronically generated blue light is an excellent first step. Don't feel guilty if you've been unaware of a device's potential danger. Each generation of moms learns new things as science evolves.

Ways to Encourage Your Baby's Development:

- Spend lots of time outside each day. Safe exposure to sunlight and fresh air is still the best environment for playtime.
- Aim for zero screen time.

Things to Remember:

I'll schedule outside playtime, so we do it.
Watching shows and staying inside a lot aren't the best choices for your development.

Chapter 154

Strike Up the Band

At 9 months, babies bang two objects together.[1]

Your baby loves to bang one object against another. For example, they may hit two items together or slam one against the floor. "Why are they banging things all the time?" you ask. Banging is another variation of cause-and-effect exploration. And while it gets annoying, especially when you have a headache, it is a typical play activity for this age.

This phase is an excellent time to set up a safe cabinet for your child to play in. Lock down all the other ones and allow exploration of what is in your child's cabinet. Ideal items include plastic cups and bowls, wooden spoons, and a few metal pots. Let them make some music and practice their drumming. Who knows? They may become a professional drummer one day.

It bears repeating that all glass-top tables and serving ware should be removed from the play area. Your child will bang anything and everything. They're too young to realize the potential danger, but you do. Ensure the place is safe.

A few musical instruments for babies may be fun. For example, a tambourine, xylophone, or drum will produce different sounds when struck. The banging action also improves your child's grip strength, which they'll need for climbing, riding toys, and future desktop work, such as writing.

Some mothers enjoy taking their babies to music-making classes. These classes are fantastic opportunities for social interactions, singing, and making music as best as each child can. You never know if you're raising a budding musician. Allow them to experience many activities and observe what they enjoy most.

Ways to Encourage Your Baby's Development:

- Babies enjoy making nonelectronic sounds—ringing bells, banging on pots, or striking the xylophone. Offer various noisemaking opportunities so they learn different sounds and tones.
- If necessary, use cotton balls in your ears or headphones to maintain your sanity. Remind yourself, once again, that this is a season. Noisy children are typical children.

Things to Remember:

I'll buy you some toy musical instruments.
I'll look around for local baby classes to see what would be fun for your age.

Chapter 155

Trying to Sing

Singing is the best way you can bring music into your child's life.[1]

Studying history makes you realize the importance of oral history and songs. Each culture has songs children learn. Most of us never forget those childhood songs, such as nursery rhymes or songs we learned at church or school. You've probably taught your baby some of your favorites.

As you sing, they may be moving and trying to sing along. Encourage them and make the song's hand motions, such as patty-cake. Whether you sing well or off-key, your baby doesn't care. Sing. Belt those words out as you do when alone in the car or shower. Sing.

Songs also make learning fun. The ABC song is one example. A quick online search will reveal many other options. Make up your own songs for bath or bedtime. Easy melodies paired with simple lyrics work well. Have fun with it.

During your child's playtimes, turn on children's music in the background. Music motivates creativity, and television shows, even with music, tend to distract from self-directed play. Try it, and you may find your child happily swaying and humming. Music is a powerful way to positively impact your little one's development.

Ways to Encourage Your Baby's Development:

- Sing and play nursery rhymes during the day. Music is a better choice than television. While many shows have music, your child may be mesmerized by the visual images and not engage in their creative play. Music by itself promotes creativity and enhances auditory memory.
- Sing songs during regular routines. Make up simple rhythms and pair them with a few words you want your child to learn, such as "Time to eat, time to eat" or "Time to sleep, time to sleep."

Things to Remember:

I'll sing to you regularly.
Your favorite song right now is

_________________________________.

Chapter 156

Where's Your Head?

The body-parts game ("Where's your nose? There it is!") is a blast for babies.[1]

It's never too early to teach your baby the names of objects and people. They may have already learned baba, mama, dada, and ball. Now is an excellent time to teach some body parts. Although they probably won't accurately point to a few—such as the nose, mouth, or head—until they're a toddler, go ahead and start.

Many parents sing "Head and Shoulders, Knees and Toes" at this age, which is excellent. However, also ask, "Where's your head? or Where's your mouth?" Many babies memorize the song, but when asked to point out a body part, they can't. Singing the song is okay. However, don't depend on it to teach your child to point to parts of their body when asked.

Babies must learn the parts of their bodies. For example, when you dress them, say, "Push your arm through the sleeve." If they don't know where their arm is, they don't understand what you're saying. They may learn what to do when getting dressed, but they aren't following your verbal command. Instead, they're imitating your actions.

Where's Your Head?

You can also ask your baby to point to your head, ears, or feet. These simple interactions teach vital language and social skills, none of which can be learned sitting alone staring at a screen. For babies and young children, face-to-face interactions are superior.

Ways to Encourage Your Baby's Development:

- During quiet times, ask your child, "Where's your head?" Then point to it or help them point to it and say, "There it is!" Babies love this game.
- When looking at picture books, ask, "Where's the doggy's nose? or "Where are the cow's eyes?" Each picture in the book has identifying characteristics you can teach, such as body parts, colors, shapes, or sounds.

Things to Remember:

The first time you pointed to your head was on

______________________________________.

If you don't enjoy these types of activities, I'll discuss this with the doctor at your next visit.

Chapter 157

Pick Me Up

By 12 months infants lift up their arms as a request to be picked up and by 6 or 7 months of age infants may already be lifting their arms up in response to the approach of a parent.[1]

By the end of a baby's first year, most already reach their arms upward when they want to be picked up. Some used to do that and now do so rarely. Sometimes, your child may seem less aware of you because they're busy exploring and playing with toys. However, when they need you, such as when they're hurt or hungry, they should resume reaching for you to pick them up.

In other cases, some children lose skills they once had. If that's your child, please talk to their doctor. Regression in previously mastered skills, such as reaching to be picked up, can signify developmental delay.

Research shows that babies learn to anticipate being picked up by looking at and leaning toward their caregivers. Unfortunately, many children with delays in social skills don't do that or do so rarely. Social engagement with others is essential for building relationships and developing communication skills. After all, if your child isn't interested in other people, they have minimal motivation to talk with them.

Pick Me Up

If your baby isn't reaching to be picked up, model the arms-up gesture as you ask, "Do you want to be picked up?" Even if they don't seem aware, keep doing it.

Ways to Encourage Your Baby's Development:

- Document your baby's milestones. Early awareness and intervention, if needed, often get your child back on track.
- Continue to model the arms-up gesture when picking them up. Implement a zero screen-time policy if you haven't already done so. Electronic entertainment is more entertaining to your child than you are. There's only one way to change that. Turn off the screens.

Things to Remember:

I'll track your milestones.
I'll adjust for prematurity, if necessary, when considering whether your development is on track.

Chapter 158

Resisting

Trying to do it all and expecting that it all can be done exactly right is a recipe for disappointment. Perfection is the enemy.[1]

When your baby pushes your helping hand away, you may feel sad or annoyed. "Why don't they want my help?" you ask yourself. "I love them and want only the best for them; besides, they aren't doing what they should, so I must offer assistance." Some of us have more difficulty allowing our children to make mistakes and get messy than others do.

Perfection is the enemy in so many venues of life. Motherhood is one of those. Suppose you are one who, like me, loves an orderly home. Giving your baby the spoon and open cup means only one thing: a big mess to clean up. Mopping the floor and bathing the baby for the umpteenth time isn't what most moms want to do.

Allow your child's imperfect attempts, so they learn. After all, do you always take advice from other seasoned mothers, even your own? If you're like me, maybe you thought *I can do it all by myself. I don't need help because I'm independent and capable.* Even so, taking care of a child, a home, and a job is a lot for anyone. Perfection is the enemy. Remember that.

Resisting

Your baby may be fighting for control, and you may be too. Pick your battles. If you fight each one, you'll run out of energy, and your child may learn to "just let you do it." But do you really want a child who cannot do for themselves?

Ways to Encourage Your Baby's Development:

- If you're on a tight schedule, build in some extra time, so your baby has time to feed themselves without being rushed.
- Let your baby help lay out tomorrow's clothes. Doing so may stop morning fights over what to wear.

Things to Remember:

I'll accept help from my friends and family when offered.
A messy house or child isn't the end of the world.

Chapter 159

Flipping Pages

Around months 12 to 14, your baby may begin to turn the pages of a book, although he'll probably grab several pages at a time.[1]

Your baby learns what they practice, so giving them sturdy books that can tolerate rough handling is recommended. Thick cardboard pages that they can grasp as they flip through the pages helps them develop fine motor skills and increases their enjoyment of books.

They may flip pages like a speed reader, pick up the book and look at it from different angles, or chew on the corners. All these behaviors are typical. They're exploring how a book feels, what it does, and how it looks and tastes.

Books with push buttons often cause children to prefer trying to push those buttons more than flipping through the pages. Get books with a push-button on each page, so they can flip through and press each one. Also buy some books without those additions if your child gets preoccupied with the buttons or touch-and-feel areas.

Most children are wiggly at this age. Expect to look only at a picture or two on each page to complete the book. Don't try to read long stories unless your child enjoys them. Additionally, paper pages, such as those found in magazines or coloring books, are easily torn. Your child will enjoy thick cardboard, cloth, or vinyl books more than flimsy ones.

Ways to Encourage Your Baby's Development:

- Allow your baby to flip the page when you look at books together. Say, "Turn the page," to prompt them.
- Looking at books should be fun. However, frequently saying "No!" or "Don't tear that!" because the book has thin pages frustrates you and your baby. Instead, use books that will hold up under a child's rough handling at this age.

Things to Remember:

The first time you turned the page in a book was on

______________________________.

I'll place family pictures in a small album for you to flip through.

Chapter 160

Baby Is Walking

Most children are able to walk alone by 11–15 months, but the rate of development is variable. Some children will fall outside the expected range and yet still walk normally in the end. Walking is considered to be delayed if it has not been achieved by 18 months.[1]

When your baby takes those first steps, you feel excitement and relief. Finally, they're upright and walking, albeit clumsily for now. But they are walking! For moms whose babies were born prematurely or have had a challenging first year, walking is an even more significant event.

Having helped thousands of babies learn to walk, I understand the struggle. Walking comes easily for some children. A few take steps as early as nine months. For others, the ones I have the most experience with, walking can sometimes seem like an unattainable milestone. And for some, it will be unreachable. But the end of your baby's first year is too soon to conclude they'll never walk.

Your baby isn't considered delayed in walking until they're eighteen months old. However, some children are late bloomers, and others have been carried or frequently contained in baby-holding equipment.

Some may have floppy bodies or weak legs. Others were born prematurely, had difficult first few months, or were often hospitalized.

Whatever your situation, if your baby isn't yet walking, don't worry. You can help them get on their feet and take steps. However, always take your concerns to their doctor. Trust your mother's instinct and get an evaluation. If it'll give you some peace of mind, do it.

Ways to Encourage Your Baby's Development:

- Encourage your baby to walk to diaper changes and the high chair.
- Allow lots of time for your baby to cruise the furniture or around the edge of the playpen. See if your baby will push a toy and walk. Baby walkers with seats aren't recommended and won't help your child learn to walk on their own.

Things to Remember:

You took your first steps on your own on

______________________________.

I'll make sure the house is safe now that you're walking.

Acknowledgments

To acknowledge everyone who helped me write and publish this book, I fear that I may have left someone out. So, if I do, please know it was an oversight and not intentional.

To all the wonderful children and families it has been my honor to help over the years, your courage and joy in the face of your struggles have taught me more than I have taught you. You inspired me to continue learning, refine my skills, and never give up.

A heartfelt thank you to my husband, Rolando, for your unwavering love and support. I couldn't have done it without you. To my sons, Sam and David, I love you and am so proud of the men you've become.

To my Word Weavers writing critique groups (Destin, Pensacola, and Nashville), I'd have quit long ago without your guidance, prayer, and advice. There really aren't words to describe what y'all mean to me.

Thank you to my editor, Denise Loock. You polished my words into a thing of beauty. To Hannah Linder, my book cover designer, you amaze me! To Hannah Linder Designs for your interior formatting, you made my manuscript finally look like the book of my dreams. Thank you!

I'd be remiss to not specifically thank Cindy Sproles and Victoria Duerstock. Cindy saw potential in this manuscript in its infancy. Victoria's coaching brought it into full maturity. Thank you both for your willingness to help an inexperienced writer who was unsure of what to do next.

And to God, Your grace amazes me. While it took three long years to get this work published, You never stopped guiding and providing. My prayer is, and has always been, that this book teaches mothers practical ways to help their babies blossom into the beautiful souls You know they are.

Section Five

Appendix

Developmental Milestones

Most babies should meet the following milestones. If your baby was born prematurely, they should meet these milestones by their adjusted age.

If your baby isn't meeting these milestones, talk to their doctor. Early identification of delays is always recommended. But it's never too late to help your child catch up.

By Three Months:

- Movement/Physical Development Milestones
  - Holds head up when on tummy
  - Moves both arms and both legs
  - Opens hands briefly
- Social/Emotional Milestones
  - Calms down when spoken to or is picked up
  - Looks at your face
  - Seems happy to see you when you walk up
  - Smiles when you talk to or smile at them
- Language/Communication Milestones

    - Makes sounds other than crying
    - Reacts to loud sounds
- Cognitive (learning, thinking, problem-solving) Milestones
    - Watches you as you move
    - Looks at a toy for several seconds

By Six Months:

- Movement/Physical Development Milestones
    - Rolls from tummy to back
    - Pushes up with straight arms when on tummy
    - Leans on hands to support self when sitting
- Social/Emotional Milestones
    - Knows familiar people
    - Likes to look at self in a mirror
    - Laughs
- Language/Communication Milestones
    - Takes turns making sounds with you
    - Blows "raspberries" (sticks tongue out and blows)
    - Makes squealing noises
- Cognitive (learning, thinking, problem-solving) Milestones
    - Puts things in their mouth to explore them
    - Reaches to grab a toy they want
    - Closes lips to show they don't want more food

By Nine Months:

- Movement/Physical Development Milestones
    - Gets to a sitting position without help
    - Moves things from one hand to the other hand
    - Uses fingers to rake food toward them
    - Sits without support
- Social/Emotional Milestones
    - Is shy, clingy, or fearful around strangers

    - Shows several facial expressions—like happy, sad, angry, and surprised
    - Looks when you call their name
    - Reacts when you leave (looks, reaches for you, or cries)
    - Smiles or laughs when you play peekaboo
- Language/Communication Milestones
    - Makes different sounds like "mamama" and "bababa"
    - Lifts arms to be picked up
- Cognitive (learning, thinking, problem-solving) Milestones
    - Looks for objects when dropped out of sight (like a spoon or toy)
    - Bangs two things together

By One Year:

- Movement/Physical Development Milestones
    - Pulls up to stand
    - Walks, holding on to furniture
    - Drinks from a cup without a lid, as you hold it
    - Picks things up between thumb and pointer finger, like small bits of food
- Social/Emotional Milestones
    - Plays games with you like patty-cake
- Language/Communication Milestones
    - Waves bye-bye
    - Calls a parent mama or dada or another special name
    - Understands no (pauses briefly or stops when you say it)
- Cognitive (Learning, thinking, problem-solving) Milestones
    - Puts something in a container, like a block in a cup
    - Looks for things they see you hide, like a toy under a blanket

Source: Centers for Disease Control and Prevention, https://www.cdc.gov/ncbddd/actearly/milestones/index.html.

Developmental Red Flags for Infants

Here are some developmental red flags that can appear between birth and one year of age. If your baby exhibits any of these, report them to your pediatrician.

Birth to 3 months

- Feeding difficulties, especially if the baby is irritable
- Prefers to turn their head to one side more than the other
- Flattening of the back or side of the head
- Prefers specific postures (back arched, head tilted, clenched fists, etc.)
- Decreased movement of one side of the body compared to the other
- Excessive arching of the back or the baby is stiff or floppy

4–6 months

- Consistent arching of the back in any position
- Keeping one or both hands clenched most of the time

- Difficulty rolling onto the side and/or staying on the side
- Consistently falling forward or extending backward when sitting (at 6 months)

7–9 MONTHS

- Scooting on the back, bunny hopping on the legs, or butt scooching instead of crawling
- Unable to get the hands together at the midline (center of the chest)
- Unable to sit without support
- Trouble bearing weight on hands or arms
- Limited desire to move, explore, or climb
- Uses one side of the body more than the other
- Sitting with legs spread wide or W-sitting

10–12 MONTHS

- Lack of desire to explore the environment
- Strong preference to use one side of the body more than the other
- Cruising along furniture in only one direction
- Consistently standing, cruising, or walking on tiptoes
- Waiting for others to do everything for them
- Struggling to grasp and release objects

Other Concerns That Cause a Higher Risk for Developmental Delays

- Difficult birth history (trauma, complications at birth, etc.)
- Low birth weight
- Mother's alcohol and substance abuse during pregnancy
- Sudden or noticeable regression in abilities

Developmental delays are common. A delay does not necessarily mean a child cannot catch up. However, experts agree that early intervention services offer the best and fastest way for a kid to meet milestones and get back on track.

If you have concerns or questions, talk to your child's doctor.

Want to know more about your baby's development? Join my Baby Support Group on Facebook.

Monthly Play Ideas for Your Baby's First Year

Play is how babies learn. Playing with your baby strengthens the emotional bond between you and your child. You'll notice that these suggestions require you to interact with your baby a lot. You will not be able to play all day, but please interact with your baby most of the day. Commit to making your home as screen-free as possible. Research shows that babies who spend time on screens are at risk for developmental delays.

Month One:

Lots of time spent skin-to-skin. Stroke and cuddle. Look into your baby's eyes, smile, and talk.

Coo, babble, sing, make silly sounds, and speak normally. Your child will love the sound of your voice.

Babies love to look at things. Black-and-white cards are great. White, red, and yellow are also colors babies enjoy. Lights are also interesting. But they may love your face the most because infants adore faces.

Newborns are easily overstimulated, so follow your child's lead. If they're tired, let them rest.

Month Two:

Soothe your baby with a calm voice. Doing so teaches them that you'll meet their needs and that you are safe. Babies sense your stress and upset emotions.

Talk, sing, coo, talk baby talk, and use your regular voice throughout the day. All of these are great for your baby's brain development.

Continue with the visual activities listed above. Also, begin offering safe toys for your child to reach for (stuffed animals, overhead mobiles, teething rattles).

Help your baby look in a mirror or use a baby-safe mirror during tummy time or side-lying play.

Lay your child on their side alongside another infant and enjoy their interactions.

Take your baby on stroller walks.

Introduce gentle yet interesting new sounds, like a purring cat, crinkling paper, or rain. Avoid electronic versions of natural sounds, as the tones are different. Natural sounds are more soothing.

Month Three:

Being responsive to your baby's babbles, laughs, or coos is crucial. Your interactions teach your child that you're reliable and predictable.

Offer hand and foot rattles. They'll enjoy making sounds themselves, which will foster more movement. Ensure the rattles are safe for mouthing!

Make funny faces, and they'll try to imitate them. Imitate the faces they make as well.

Babies respond more slowly than adults. So, give them time.

Offer music with a strong beat. Clap your hands or tap your baby's feet to the beat.

Introduce sturdy picture books, preferably one or two pictures per page. Point and name objects, animals, or people pictured.

Allow your baby to experience different textures, such as a soft blanket, a rough towel, or a slick floor. Doing so helps your baby get used to various sensations.

During bath time, blow bubbles.

Month Four:

Begin playing peekaboo. By month four, your child will learn about object permanence, which means knowing that an object or person is still there even when they disappear.

Continue with mirror play, mobiles, activity boards, and teething rings.

Continue introducing sounds, like tapping a drum, ringing a bell, or clicking your tongue.

Hold up picture books and point to and name the objects, animals, or people pictured. Say "turn" when you turn the page.

Month Five:

Begin more community outings, such as going to a playground, to meet other babies.

Offer baths as a play activity. Splashing is fun!

Begin rolling balls. Your child will enjoy watching them roll. Doing so improves visual tracking skills, which are vital for many upcoming milestones.

Continue with lots of playtime on the floor (use a playmat).

When your baby begins to pass a toy from one hand to the other, offer them teething rings or lightweight objects to use.

Allow your baby to spend a few minutes in swings or bouncy chairs. Visit with them instead of turning on the TV or tablet.

At this age, your child may begin rolling over. Provide a safe space on the floor for lots of practice.

Continue cooing, babbling, singing, and speaking in your natural voice throughout the day.

Try whispering to see if they hear and respond. Sing their name and see if they turn toward you.

Month Six:

Cover a favorite toy with a lightweight blanket or towel. Ask your baby, "Where did it go?" and see if they try to pull the blanket away. This game is a variation of the peekaboo game, where your tot is learning about object permanence.

If your baby enjoys a baby swing, say "hello" as they swing toward you and "goodbye" as they move away.

When you pick up your baby's toys, name them—block, ball, or baby. This activity teaches your child the names of the toys and enhances their vocabulary.

Begin pointing to and naming body parts. Babies love this game, especially the nose, eye, mouth, and ears. You can also do this while looking in a mirror.

At this age, babies enjoy hand play, such as patty-cake and the motions for the song "The Wheels on the Bus."

When your baby makes a sound or funny face, imitate them. Make it fun!

Describe objects using their color. "Look at the red ball!" or "She's wearing a pink hat." Doing this expands your baby's vocabulary to include nouns and adjectives.

Place toys around your child during floor time to encourage them to move around and reach for them.

Babies love everyday objects! Begin offering safe items to explore, such as wooden spoons, plastic bowls, or plastic measuring spoons.

Month Seven:

While your child is on their tummy, stand up and make noises or shake a favorite toy to get them to look up and push up on their hands.

Continue playing peekaboo. Vary it by hiding a toy under a pillow, blanket, or bucket and encouraging your baby to find it.

Ask your tot questions during conversations and respond to their answers (even if they're nonsensical). The point is to teach your child that you're listening and engaging.

Food is a game at this age. Let your baby grab food with their fists and shove it toward their mouth. They're not trying to make a mess; they're exploring, and a mess will result.

Lay out objects they recognize. Ask, "Where's the book?" or "Where's your ball?" Praise them when they're correct, but don't chastise them for their mistakes.

Month Eight:

At this age, babies love dropping, banging, and tossing items. It's a phase, but it can be exasperating.

Make funny faces, shake your head, or make funny sounds. Your baby is learning to imitate motor actions. Imitation of motor actions is a crucial phase in cognitive development.

Provide an empty bottom drawer for them to open and close. (Be careful they don't pinch their fingers or climb in and topple the furniture.)

Create an easy obstacle course for your baby if they're crawling or scooting.

Hide behind a door and make your baby push it open to find and see you. This game is another version of peekaboo, and children at this age love it.

Toss a ball in the air and make a silly sound when it hits the floor.

Play chasing games. You can crawl behind them or in front.

Stack blocks and then show your baby how to knock them down.

Present easy shape puzzles and interlocking toys. Put them together and take them apart again.

Read to your child. It's one of the best things you can do. Hearing new words and sounds helps develop their communication skills.

Month Nine:

Learn the concepts of inside and outside using a large cardboard box. You can cut a door in it.

At a park or beach, show your baby a brightly colored baby-safe object, like a rubber ball. Then, bury the toy under some sand. Ask, "Where did it go?"

Place objects around your baby that you know they'll recognize. Then ask, "Where's the spoon? or "Where's the bucket?"

Drop, throw, or bang just about anything to see what happens. This idea explores cause and effect.

Month Ten:

Teach the parts of a doll or stuffed animal, including hair, eyes, ears, and toes. Name the parts aloud.

Give them a bucket of toys and let them dump it out and fill it up again. You can also give them stacking toys, like rings and cups.

Sing songs that encourage finger games and have a lot of repetition, like "The Wheels on the Bus" or "Itsy Bitsy Spider."

Push a small car or truck along the floor. After a while, they'll learn to let go, allowing the car to roll by itself.

Talk to them on a real or play phone. They'll learn the fun of conversation.

Go outside. Gather leaves, twigs, or toys in a pail.

Put a small toy inside a paper bag or box. Doing so teaches an understanding of inside and outside.

Build a tower of blocks. Watch them as they fall.

Bang and clap using sticks, spoons, and other utensils.

Month Eleven:

Bounce on a mattress that is on the floor. Prevent falls, of course.

Lie on the floor and encourage your child to crawl back and forth over your back.

Play with sand or water. Babies love dumping and filling buckets or bowls.

Stand your baby on their knees or feet and rock slowly to music together.

Continue making funny faces and sounds to see if your baby imitates them.

Clap hands—both your own and your baby's. They will love playing new clapping games.

Ask your baby to get simple objects for you to use by naming them.

Month Twelve:

Cruise along the furniture or walk with your baby, singing happily to make them smile.

Take turns doing things like stacking blocks and knocking them down.

Continue talking and singing to their heart's delight.

Encourage fine motor development with finger games and songs like "Itsy Bitsy Spider" and "Baby Shark."

Enjoy imitative play. Use phones, kitchen utensils, tools, dolls, cars, and animals. Pretend to talk on the phone, feed the stuffed bear, or stir the stew. Encourage them to imitate.

Your baby may enjoy purposeful play, like using a plastic hammer to pound pegs into a hole.

Point and name different objects and see if they try to reach for or name them.

Get easy-to-hold board books and cloth books, and continue reading.

Make different animal noises as you point to the animals in picture books or play with toy animal figures.

Place circular objects, such as cereal, on a thick pipe cleaner and see if your baby wants to try to do that too. This is a great activity to strengthen pincer grasp.

Do everyday routines, like brushing your hair and folding wash-cloths, and see if they want to try to do it too.

Additional Reading

Nicolas Kardaras. *Glow Kids: How Screen Addiction Is Hijacking Our Kids—and How to Break the Trance*. London: Macmillan, 2016.

Mary S. Kurcinka. *Raising Your Spirited Baby: A Breakthrough Guide to Thriving When Your Baby Is More ... Alert and Intense and Struggles to Sleep*. New York: William Morrow, 2020.

Notes

1. Love at First Sight

1. "Frank A. Clark Quotes," BrainyQuote, accessed September 19, 2022, https://www.brainyquote.com/quotes/frank_a_clark_106520.

2. First Breath

1. "Your first breath took ours away" | New Baby Quotes," Pinterest, accessed September 19, 2022, https://www.pinterest.com/pin/keegan--167125836150732580/.

3. What's in a Name?

1. Personal interview, Florida, 2019.

4. Looks Like

1. Himanshi Bahuguna, "When Your Baby Is a Mini-me of Dad, but You Did all the Heavy Lifting," Motherly, last modified on April 9, 2025, https://www.mother.ly/news/viral-trending/viral-tiktok-when-your-baby-looks-like-dad/.

5. Your Baby's Skin

1. "Why Baby's Sense of Smell Is Important," Pathways.org | Tools to Maximize Your Child's Development, accessed July 19, 2025, https://pathways.org/babys-sense-of-smell.

6. Mother's Milk

1. "Recommendations and Benefits," Centers for Disease Control and Prevention, last modified July 9, 2021, https://www.cdc.gov/nutrition/infantandtoddlernutrition/breastfeeding/recommendations-benefits.html.

7. Overwhelmed

1. "40 Inspiring Quotes About Being a Mother." The Church of Jesus Christ of Latter-day Saints, accessed July19, 2025, https://www.churchofjesuschrist.org/comeuntochrist/belong/family/40-quotes-about-motherhood.

2. "Baby Blues," American Pregnancy Association, last modified December 9, 2021, https://americanpregnancy.org/healthy-pregnancy/first-year-of-life/baby-blues/.

8. TONGUE-TIED

1. Heidi Murkoff and Sharon Mazel, *What To Expect The 1st Year*, 3rd Edition, What to Expect, 2018.

9. WHITE NOISE

1. Kristeen Cherney, "The Pros and Cons of Using White Noise to Put Babies to Sleep," Healthline, accessed July 28, 2022, https://www.healthline.com/health/parenting/white-noise-for-babies#importance-of-sleep.

10. THE NOSE KNOWS

1. "Women's Superior Sense of Smell May Be Due to More Brain Cells, Study Says," Fox News, last modified February 1, 2015, https://www.foxnews.com/health/womens-superior-sense-of-smell-may-be-due-to-more-brain-cells-study-says.

11. TEARS

1. Sarah Bradley, "When Do Babies Start Crying Tears?" Healthline, July 31, 2020, https://www.healthline.com/health/baby/when-do-babies-get-tears.

12. SOLE CARE

1. Jonathan Boxall, "Your Feet Were Made for Walking," Osteo&Physio, January 8, 2019, https://osteoandphysio.co.uk/your-feet-were-made-for-walking/.

13. GRIEF

1. "A Quote from *A Grief Observed*," Goodreads, accessed July 28, 2022, https://www.goodreads.com/quotes/649744-no-one-ever-told-me-that-grief-felt-so-like.

14. ROCKABYE BABY

1. "Rock-a-bye Baby," Wikipedia Foundation, last modified November 8, 2005, https://en.wikipedia.org/wiki/Rock-a-bye_Baby.

15. RUNNING ON EMPTY

1. J. Browne, "Running on Empty," *Running on Empty*. Asylum Records, 1978.

16. Lift Your Eyes

1. Isaiah 40:26 (NIV).

17. Lay Down

1. "I Just Want to Lay Down on a Beach, Let the Sun Hit My Face and Forget About Absolutely Every... | Inspirational Quotes Motivation, Beach Quotes, Inspirational Quotes," Pinterest, accessed September 20, 2022, https://www.pinterest.com/pin/82542605653855645/.

18. Just a Whisper

1. Deborah L. Bennett, "Understanding the Stages of Baby Babble," SentinelSource, last modified May 18, 2012, https://www.sentinelsource.com/parent_express/pregnancy_babies/understanding-the-stages-of-baby-babble/article_611d18f4-a11d-11e1-8120-0019bb2963f4.html#:~:text=In%20the%20Expansion%20Stage%2C%20beginning,Laughter%20emerges%20at%20this%20time.

19. I Hear You

1. "Hearing," *The Merriam-Webster Dictionary*, Merriam-Webster, accessed August 16, 2025, https://www.merriam-webster.com/dictionary/hearing.

20. Going Without Sleep

1. "Dr. Seuss Quote: "Sleep is Like the Unicorn—It is Rumored to Exist, but I Doubt I Will See Any" | Inspirational Quotes on Beautiful Wallpapers, QuoteFancy, accessed July 7, 2025, https://quotefancy.com/quote/795850/Dr-Seuss-Sleep-is-like-the-unicorn-it-is-rumored-to-exist-but-I-doubt-I-will-see-any.
2. Amy R. Wolfson and Kathryn A. Lee, *The Woman's Book of Sleep: A Complete Resource Guide*, New Harbinger Publications, 2001.

21. Fussy

1. Catherine Pearson, "Why Are Some Babies SO Much Harder Than Others?" HuffPost, last modified September 14, 2016, https://www.huffpost.com/entry/why-are-some-babies-so-much-harder-than-others_n_57cec79be4b078581f13e82e.

22. Fisted Hands

1. Kimberly Zapata, "Baby Clenching Fists? There's Probably a Simple Explanation," Healthline, accessed August 1, 2022, https://www.healthline.com/health/baby/baby-clenching-fist#when-does-it-stop.

23. First Smile

1. "Emotional and Social Development, Ages 1 to 12 Months," University of Michigan Health | Michigan Medicine, accessed August 1, 2022, https://www.uofmhealth.org/health-library/ue5463#:~:text=Around%202%20months%20of%20age,familiar%20caregivers%20than%20for%20strangers.

24. Feeding Troubles

1. "Breastfeeding," HealthyChildren, accessed August 1, 2022, https://www.healthychildren.org/English/ages-stages/baby/breastfeeding/Pages/default.aspx.

25. Eyes on Me

1. Hebrews 12:2 (NIV).

26. Different Cries

1. "Decoding Baby Crying: 8 Types of Crying You Might Hear," Mom Loves Best, last modified June 15, 2025, https://momlovesbest.com/decoding-baby-crying.

27. Crossed Eyes

1. Donna Christiano, "Why Do Babies Go Cross Eyed, and Will It Go Away?" Healthline, June 16, 2020, https://www.healthline.com/health/baby/cross-eyed-baby#symptoms.

28. Born for a Purpose

1. Ephesians 2:10 (NIV).

29. Being Held

1. "What Is Self-Soothing? Learn About This Important Social-Emotional Tool," Pathways, last modified May 25, 2022, https://pathways.org/self-soothing/.

30. Another Load

1. "Laundry Facts Speak Volumes About Family Habits," Chron, last modified August 18, 2011, https://www.chron.com/life/article/Laundry-facts-speak-volumes-about-family-habits-2091022.php.

31. A Little Extra

1. "Down Syndrome: MedlinePlus Genetics," MedlinePlus | Health Information from the National Library of Medicine, accessed September 19, 2022, https://medline plus.gov/genetics/condition/down-syndrome/.

32. Black and White

1. "Your Newborn's Hearing, Vision, and Other Senses," Nemours Kidhealth, accessed August 5, 2022, https://kidhealth.org/en/parents/sensenewborn.html.

33. Something Is Wrong

1. Tracey Harrington McCoy, "Parent's Intuition Is Real and Here's Why You Should Trust It," Parents, last modified February 14, 2023, https://www.parents.com/parent ing/moms/mothers-intuition-is-real-and-heres-why-you-should-trust-it/.

34. Born Too Early

1. Preterm Birth," Maternal Infant Health, last modified May 20, 2024, https://www.cdc.gov/maternal-infant-health/preterm-birth/?CDC_AAref_Val=https://www.cdc.gov/reproductivehealth/maternalinfanthealth/pretermbirth.htm.

35. Beware of Containers

1. "Container Baby Syndrome: How Equipment Can Hinder a Child's Development," Nationwide Children's Hospital, last modified October 23, 2018, https://www.nation widechildrens.org/family-resources-education/700childrens/2018/10/container-baby-syndrome#:~:text=Container%20Baby%20Syndrome%20may%20be,of%20movement%20known%20as%20plagiocephaly.

36. Staying Warm

1. Keeping Your Baby Warm," Stanford Medicine | Children's Health, accessed August 8, 2022, https://www.stanfordchildrens.org/en/topic/default?id=warmth-and-temperature-regulation-90-P02425.

37. Pat and Bat

1. Jennifer Kelly Geddes, "When Do Babies Start Reaching?" What to Expect, last modified August 14, 2017, https://www.whattoexpect.com/first-year/reaching/.

38. Both Ends of the Bed

1. "Flat Head Syndrome (Positional Plagiocephaly)," Nemours Kidhealth, accessed August 5, 2022, https://kidhealth.org/en/parents/positional-plagiocephaly.html.

39. Feel the Rhythm

1. "Sense of Rhythm," Merriam–Webster, accessed August 5, 2022, https://www.merriam-webster.com/dictionary/sense%20of%20rhythm.

40. Wait and See

1. "Wait and See Quotes by Wendy Pope," Goodreads, accessed August 8, 2022, https://www.goodreads.com/work/quotes/48123691-wait-and-see-finding-peace-in-god-s-pauses-and-plans.

41. Looking at Hands

1. His little hands stole my heart ... and his little feet ran aways with it | Baby Feet Quotes," Pinterest, accessed August 8, 2022, https://www.pinterest.com/pin/406801778840329060/.

42. Mother's Voice

1. "Hearing & Making Sounds: Your Baby's Milestones," HealthyChildren.org, accessed August 8, 2022, https://www.healthychildren.org/English/ages-stages/baby/Pages/Hearing-and-Making-Sounds.aspx.

43. Oohs and Aahs

1. Amy Cuevas Schroeder,"10 Funny Quotes About Motherhood, Parenting, and Raising Kids," The Midst, last modified September 2, 2021, https://the-midst.com/funny-mom-quotes/.

44. Peekaboo

1. "Peekaboo," Wikipedia Foundation, last modified September 28, 2005, https://en.wikipedia.org/wiki/Peekaboo.

45. Who's That Baby?

1. Dan Puglisi, "Reflecting on Babies and Mirror Play," First Things First, last modified May 1, 2022, https://www.firstthingsfirst.org/first-things/reflecting-on-babies-and-mirror-play/.

46. Where's Your Nose?

1. "Knowing Yourself Is the Beginning of All Wisdom – Aristotle," Goodreads, accessed August 18, 2025, https://www.goodreads.com/quotes/3102-knowing-yourself-is-the-beginning-of-all-wisdom.

47. Learning to Calm Down

1. "Motherhood Quotes (1686 Quotes)," Goodreads, accessed August11, 2022, https://www.goodreads.com/quotes/tag/motherhood.

48. Kicking the Kitty

1. Linda Rogers, "When Do Babies Start Playing with Toys?" What to Expect, accessed August 15, 2025, https://www.whattoexpect.com/first-year/milestones/when-babies-start-playing-with-toys.

49. Watching It Fall

1. Shelby Stewart, "Why Babies Drop Objects and What to Do," Metro Parent | Detroit and Ann Arbor Metro, July 22, 2022, https://www.metroparent.com/parenting/advice/why-babies-drop-objects-and-what-to-do/.

50. Baby Laughs

1. Kerry Weiss, "When Do Babies Start Laughing?" What to Expect, last modified August 8, 2017, https://www.whattoexpect.com/first-year/first-laugh/.

51. I Know You

1. Mahak Arora, "When Do Babies Recognize Their Mother, Father, & Other Familiar People?" FirstCry Parenting, last modified July 10, 2023, https://parenting.firstcry.com/articles/when-do-babies-recognize-their-mother-father-and-other-familiar-people/.

52. Time to Pivot

1. "Lumiere Children's Therapy Chicago: Mastering Gross Motor Milestones," Lumiere Children's Therapy, last modified May 15, 2019, https://www.lumierechild.com/lumiere-childrens-therapy/2019/5/15/lumiere-childrens-therapy-chicago-mastering-gross-motor-milestones.

53. Arms Up

1. Rachel Rief Ellis, "Milestones for Your Baby's First Year," WebMD, last modified June 13, 2017, https://www.webmd.com/parenting/baby/baby-first-year-milestones.

54. Reaching and Grasping

1. Allison Banfield, "Encouraging Mom Quotes," Proud Happy Mama, last modified July 14, 2022, https://proudhappymama.com/21-encouraging-mom-quotes-every-mother-needs-to-read/.

55. Praying Hands

1. Wendi McKenna, DPT, PCS, and C/NDT, "Developmental Red Flags for Infants," The Inspired Treehouse, last modified April 12, 2022, https://theinspiredtreehouse.com/common-developmental-red-flags-infants/.

56. Shake, Rattle, and Roll

1. "Shake, Rattle and Roll," Fandom | Muppet Wiki, accessed September 20, 2022, https://muppet.fandom.com/wiki/Shake,_Rattle_and_Roll.

57. Into the Mouth

1. Noreen Iftikhar, "Baby Mouthing—AKA Why Do Babies Put Everything in Their Mouths?" Healthline, accessed August 15, 2022, https://www.healthline.com/health/baby/baby-mouthing.

58. Hand to Hand

1. Ellis, "Milestones for Your Baby's First Year," WebMD.

59. Babbling

1. Ellis, "Milestones for Your Baby's First Year," WebMD.

60. Rolling Over

1. Ellis, "Milestones for Your Baby's First Year," WebMD.

61. Sitting Up

1. "Jane Clayson Quotes," BrainyQuote, accessed August 15, 2022, https://www.brainyquote.com/authors/jane-clayson-quotes.

62. Sucking on Toes

1. Boxhall, "Your Feet Were Made for Walking," Osteo&Physio.

63. Splash Time

1. "Vision Development: Newborn to 12 Months," American Academy of Ophthalmology, last modified February 1, 2022, https://www.aao.org/eye-health/tips-prevention/baby-vision-development-first-year.

64. Bouncing

1. WebMD Editorial Contributor, "When Can a Baby Use a Jumper Toy?" WebMD, last modified March 22, 2021, https://www.webmd.com/baby/when-can-a-baby-use-a-jumper-toy.

65. Clap, Clap

1. Sarah Bradley, "Cue the Applause: When Do Babies Start Clapping," Healthline, March 23, 2020, https://www.healthline.com/health/baby/when-do-babies-clap.

66. Holding the Bottle

1. Lara Heard, "When Do Babies Hold Their Own Bottles?" What to Expect, last modified June 29, 2022, https://www.whattoexpect.com/first-year/bottle-feeding/when-do-babies-hold-bottles.

67. Call My Name

1. Ashley Marcin, "When Do Babies Know Their Name?" Healthline, July 22, 2021, https://www.healthline.com/health/baby/when-do-babies-know-their-name.

68. Lazy Baby

1. "My Baby Isn't Lazy, and Neither Is Yours," The Motherload, last modified January 15, 2018, https://the-motherload.co.uk/my-baby-isnt-lazy-and-neither-is-yours/.

69. Can't Lie Down

1. "90% of Parenting Is Just Thinking About When You Can Lie Down Again! | Parenting," Pinterest, accessed August 19, 2022, https://www.pinterest.com/pin/90-of-parenting-is-just-thinking-about-when-you-can-lie-down-again--165366617553877643/.

70. Pureed Foods

1. "Solid Foods: How to Get Your Baby Started," Mayo Clinic, last modified October 27, 2021, https://www.mayoclinic.org/healthy-lifestyle/infant-and-toddler-health/in-depth/healthy-baby/art-20046200.

71. Where's Baby?

1. Aivaras Kaziukonis and Justé Kairyté-Barkauskiené, "127 Funny Mom Quotes That Any Parent Will Find Relatable," Bored Panda, last modified March 15, 2022, https://www.boredpanda.com/funny-mom-quotes/?utm_source=google&utm_medium=organic&utm_campaign=organic.

72. Don't Drop That

1. Shelby Stewart, "Why Babies Drop Objects and What to Do," MetroParent, July 22, 2022, https://www.metroparent.com/parenting/advice/why-babies-drop-objects-and-what-to-do/.

73. Oh No!

1. "Language Milestones: 0 to 12 Months," Healthline, accessed August 19, 2022, https://www.healthline.com/health/baby/language-milestones-0-to-12-months.

74. Blowing Raspberries

1. WebMD Editorial Contributors, "Why Does a Baby Blow Raspberries?" WebMD, last modified March 14, 2021, https://www.webmd.com/baby/why-does-a-baby-blow-raspberries.

75. Sleeping All Night

1. Maria Masters, "When Will My Baby Sleep Through the Night? Here's the Scoop," What to Expect, August 13, 2025, https://www.whattoexpect.com/first-year/sleeping-through-the-night.aspx.

76. WAVING BYE-BYE

1. Team Lovevery, "When Do Babies Wave?" Lovevery, last modified April 19, 2022, https://lovevery.com/community/blog/child-development/when-do-babies-wave/.

77. PUSHING UP

1. Kandis Lake, R.N., "When Do Babies Push Up on Their Hands?" BabyCenter, last modified October 8, 2015, https://www.babycenter.com/baby/baby-development/should-i-worry-that-my-4-month-old-cant-do-mini-pushups-yet_2077.

78. GOING FOR A RIDE

1. "It's Science: This is Why Your Baby Always Falls Asleep in the Car," Motherly, last modified October 14, 2021, https://www.mother.ly/life/why-do-car-rides-put-babies-to-sleep/.

79. HAVING A BALL

1. "The Importance of Ball Play in Childhood Development," Crocodile Creek Australia, last modified February 18, 2021, https://crocodilecreekaus.com.au/blogs/news/the-importance-of-ball-play-in-childhood-development.

80. SMALL TALK

1. "What Do I Talk to My Baby About?" the *HealthPartners* blog, last modified February 24, 2022, https://www.healthpartners.com/blog/talk-to-my-baby/.

81. STRANGER DANGER

1. Jennifer Kelly Geddes, "How to Deal with Stranger Anxiety," What to Expect, last modified October 13, 2021, https://www.whattoexpect.com/toddler-behavior/toddler-stranger-anxiety.aspx.

82. WANT A CRACKER?

1. Colleen de Bellefonds, "When Will My Baby's Teeth Come In? Check Our Baby Teeth Chart," What to Expect, last modified May 5, 2016, https://www.whattoexpect.com/first-year/teething/order-of-baby-teeth-tooth-chart/.

83. THAT'S HEAVY

1. "30 Funny Weekend Quotes Cause Cheers to the Freaking Weekend | The Funny Beaver | Funny Weekend Quotes, Weekend Quotes, Quotes About Motherhood,"

Pinterest, last modified August 7, 2020, https://www.pinterest.com/pin/531354456047190614/?mt=login.

84. DADA

1. Deborah MacNamara, “No Worries, Mama: Saying ‘Dada’ First Actually Means You & Baby Are Super Bonded,” Motherly, last modified February 25, 2025, https://www.mother.ly/parenting/no-worries-mama-saying-dada-first-actually-means-you-baby-are-super-bonded/.

85. SAY MAMA!

1. Brenda Kosciuk, “72 Baby Quotes For Mom That Express Pure Love,” Paper Heart Family, last modified June 23, 2022, https://www.paperheartfamily.com/baby-quotes-new-moms/.

86. OPEN AND CLOSE

1. “Making Space for Your Baby,” Milk Planet, December 17, 2021, https://milkplanet.com.my/making-space-for-your-baby.

87. COMBAT CRAWLING

1. “Learning to Crawl,” Pregnancy Birth and Baby, last modified May 18, 2022, https://www.pregnancybirthbaby.org.au/learning-to-crawl.

88. W-SITTING

1. Rebecca Bazzoni, “What Is W-Sitting?” Joe’s Kids, accessed July 8, 2025, https://www.joes-kids.org/blog/w-sitting-why-you-should-be-concerned/.

89. STEADY SITTING

1. “When Your Baby Will Sit Up—With Your Help and Alone,” What to Expect, last modified September 30, 2015, https://www.whattoexpect.com/first-year/sit-up/.

90. GETTING INTO SITTING

1. “When Your Baby Will Sit Up—With Your Help and Alone,” What to Expect.

91. SITTING TO CRAWLING

1. “When Do Babies Start Crawling?” What to Expect, last modified August 24, 2015. https://www.whattoexpect.com/first-year/crawling/.

92. Clapping Hands

1. Sarah Bradley, "When Do Babies Clap? Plus, How to Encourage This Milestone," Healthline, accessed August 18, 2022, https://www.healthline.com/health/baby/when-do-babies-clap.

93. Let's Play Peekaboo

1. Linda Rogers, "When Do Babies Play Peekaboo," What to Expect, last modified February 6, 2018, https://www.whattoexpect.com/first-year/peek-a-boo/.

94. Baby on the Move

1. "Why Baby Walkers Can Put Your Child in Danger," University Hospitals, last modified September 24, 2018, https://www.uhhospitals.org/Healthy-at-UH/articles/2018/09/why-baby-walkers-can-put-your-child-in-danger.

95. Getting into Stuff

1. "100+ Funny Baby Quotes That Will Make You Giggle." Scary Mommy, accessed August 29, 2022, https://www.scarymommy.com/funny-baby-quotes.

96. Did You Call?

1. Kerry Weiss, "When Do Babies Recognize and Respond to Their Name?" What to Expect, last modified October 30, 2015, https://www.whattoexpect.com/first-year/understand-words/.

97. Moving and Grooving

1. Marygrace Taylor, "Musical Play for Babies and Toddlers," What to Expect, last modified April 12, 2017, https://www.whattoexpect.com/first-year/playtime/music-baby-development/.

98. Don't Leave Me

1. "I Don't Need a Big, Fancy Vacation. I'd Be Happy with a Trip to the Bathroom by Myself. | Mommy Humor, Mommy Memes, Funny Quotes," Pinterest, accessed August 29, 2022, https://www.pinterest.com/pin/137500594843595511/.

99. Pulling Off Socks

1. "Why Do Babies Take Off Their Socks?," Fairy Good Mommy, accessed August 29, 2022, https://www.fairygoodmommy.com/why-do-babies-take-off-their-socks/.

100. Timber!

1. "The Importance of Destructive Play for Babies and Toddlers," Inspiration Laboratories, last modified April 15, 2019, https://inspirationlaboratories.com/importance-of-destructive-play/.

101. For Me?

1. Colleen Beck, "Tear Paper for Fine Motor Skills," The OT Toolbox, last modified August 31, 2021, https://www.theottoolbox.com/torn-paper-art-awesome-fine-motor/.

102. Up and Down

1. "How to Help Babies and Toddlers When They Fall," Pathways, last modified May 25, 2022, https://pathways.org/baby-falling/.

103. Crawling Under

1. Anna Lacey, "Peek-a-boo: A Window on Baby's Brain," BBC News, last modified March 11, 2014, https://www.bbc.com/news/health-24553877.

104. Pulling Mommy Over

1. "Tug of War," Wikipedia Foundation, last modified June 23, 2025, https://en.wikipedia.org/wiki/Tug_of_war#:~:text=The%20origins%20of%20-tug%20of,each%20end%20of%20the%20rope.

105. Shake It, Baby!

1. Rebecca Grant, "Born to Dance: Why Music Is So Good for Babies," Medibank | New Parents, last modified December 9, 2018, https://www.medibank.com.au/livebetter/families/new-parents/born-to-dance-why-music-is-so-good-for-babies/.

106. Clean Out the Basket

1. Samantha Lawler, "50 Funny Mom Quotes That Will Make You Laugh Out Loud," Woman's Day, last modified March 31, 2023, https://www.womansday.com/relationships/family-friends/g35801745/funny-mom-quotes/?slide=7.

107. All Done!

1. Karen Robock, "Baby Sign Language: The Only 8 Signs You Need to Teach Your

Baby," Today's Parent | Baby Development, last modified April 27, 2023, https://www.todaysparent.com/baby/baby-development/baby-sign-language-first-signs/.

108. Baby Wants Milk

1. Joanne Lewsley, "My 10-month-old Only Wants Milk. Should I Worry?" BabyCentre UK, last modified October 22, 2024, https://www.babycentre.co.uk/x554992/my-10-month-old-only-wants-milk-should-i-worry.

109. Hat Shopping

1. First Word Projects, "Baby and Toddler Milestones: 16 Actions with Objects by 16 Months," Reading Rockets, last modified June 10, 2020, https://www.readingrockets.org/article/baby-and-toddler-milestones-16-actions-objects-16-months.

110. Not Enough Hands

1. "You're Doing Good | Quotable Quotes, Quotes, Inspirational Words," Pinterest, last modified October 5, 2014, https://www.pinterest.com/pin/10273905376093436/?mt=login.

111. Put It In

1. Putting Away and into Containers: Why Voluntary Release Is Important to Baby's Development," ADAM & Mila, last modified April 13, 2016, https://www.adam-mila.com/milestones/fine-motor-skills/put-in-take-out/.

112. Mommy Said No!

1. Maria Masters, "Can You Teach a Baby Discipline?" What to Expect, last modified March 4, 2015, https://www.whattoexpect.com/baby-behavior/teaching-discipline.aspx.

113. What's That Sound?

1. "Language Milestones: 0 to 12 Months," Healthline, accessed August 19, 2022, https://www.healthline.com/health/baby/language-milestones-0-to-12-months.

114. Fist Bump

1. "Milestones: 8-12 Months: Physical Development," Nabta Health, accessed July 8, 2025, https://nabtahealth.com/article/milestones-8-12-months-physical-development/.

115. Mommy Kiss It

1. "Kissing Your Kid's 'Boo-Boos' Really Does Make Them Heal Faster, Says Science," CafeMom, accessed September 4, 2022, https://cafemom.com/parenting/206246-kissing_saliva_heals_kid_wounds_study.

116. Baby Faces

1. Jennifer Adaeze Okwerekwu, "Your Baby Isn't As Clever As You Think," STAT, last modified May 5, 2016, https://www.statnews.com/2016/05/05/newborn-baby-imitate/.

117. Are You Sad?

1. Ayelet Marinovich, MA, CCC-SLP, "Helping Infants & Toddlers Understand Feelings," Learn With Less, last modified September 27, 2019, https://learnwithless.com/podcast/labelling-emotions/.

118. Over My Leg

1. "Why Is Baby Crawling On Hands & Knees Important for Development?" Imagine Pediatric Therapy, the *Imagine Pediatric Therapy* blog, last modified March 26, 2021, https://www.imaginepeds.com/why-is-baby-crawling-on-hands-knees-important-for-development/.

119. Let's Swing

1. Cat Bowen, "Why Does Your Baby Hate Their Swing?" Romper, June 5, 2017, https://www.romper.com/p/why-does-my-baby-hate-their-swing-expert-weighs-in-62043.

120. Baby Standers

1. The Best Way to Use Baby Seats and Activity Centers, According to a Pediatric PT," The Everymom, last modified August 9, 2022, https://theeverymom.com/baby-activity-center-seat-bouncer-jumper-walker/.

121. Don't Want

1. "Infants: 16 Gestures by 16 Months," The Warren Center | Non-profit Organization in Richardson, Texas, last modified October 7, 2021, https://thewarrencenter.org/help-information/communication/infants-16-gestures-by-16-months/.

122. WAVING HELLO

1. Team Lovevery, "When Do Babies Wave?" Lovevery.

123. HOLDING THE SPOON

1. Fingers, Spoons, Forks, and Cups," Centers for Disease Control and Prevention (CDC) | Infant and Toddler Nutrition, October 17, 2024, https://www.cdc.gov/infant-toddler-nutrition/mealtime/fingers-spoons-forks-and-cups.html?CDC_AAref_Val=https://www.cdc.gov/nutrition/infantandtoddlernutrition/mealtime/fingers-spoons-forks-cups.html.

124. PULLING TO STANDING

1. "Take a Stand! How to Help Baby Stand on Their Own," Pathways.org., last modified May 25, 2022, https://pathways.org/help-baby-stand-on-their-own/.

125. PINCER GRASP

1. WebMD Editorial Contributors, "What to Know About Pincer Grasp," WebMD, last modified May 6, 2021, https://www.webmd.com/parenting/baby/what-to-know-pincer-grasp.

126. WHERE DID IT GO?

1. "Searching for Hidden Objects: Babies and Toddlers," Educatall, last modified November 10, 2016, https://www.educatall.com/page/1098/Searching-for-hidden-objects.html.

127. GIVE IT TO ME

1. "This Perfectly Sums Up Eating out with Kids! Haha! | Parents Quotes Funny, Funny Mom Quotes, Motherhood Funny," Pinterest, accessed September 8, 2022, https://www.pinterest.com/pin/784681935048128254/.

128. A CLIMBER

1. Harvy Karp, MD, FAAP, "When Will Your Baby Start to Climb?" the *Happiest Baby* blog, last modified November 22, 2021, https://www.happiestbaby.com/blogs/baby/when-do-babies-start-climbing.

129. PUSHING THE FURNITURE

1. "Top 50 Funny Mom Quotes for Mother's Day," Amanda Seghetti, last modified May 26, 2021, https://www.amandaseghetti.com/top-10-funny-quotes-moms/.

130. MAKING MOMMY LAUGH

1. "How Your Baby's Sense of Humor Develops—And What You Can Do to Boost It," BBC | CBeebies Parenting, last modified June 21, 2022, https://www.bbc.co.uk/tiny-happy-people/articles/zjtsvk7.

131. WATCH ME

1. Marygrace Taylor, "When Can Babies and Toddlers Watch TV?" What to Expect, last modified January 28, 2015, https://www.whattoexpect.com/toddler-discipline/toddlers-and-tv.aspx.

132. COMFORTING OTHERS

1. Peter Gray, PhD, "Infants' Instincts to Help, Share, and Comfort," Psychology Today, last modified September 30, 2018, https://www.psychologytoday.com/us/blog/freedom-learn/201809/infants-instincts-help-share-and-comfort.

133. ROLL IT BACK

1. Wendy Wisner, "The Ages and Stages of Play," Parents, last modified July 2, 2023, https://www.parents.com/toddlers-preschoolers/development/growth/ages-and-stages-of-play/.

134. TURN IT

1. First Word Projects, "Baby and Toddler Milestones: 16 Actions with Objects by 16 Months," Reading Rockets.

135. FLIP THE SWITCH

1. Vanessa LoBue, PhD, "Why Children Like Repetition, and How It Helps Them Learn," Psychology Today, last modified July 10, 2019, https://www.psychologytoday.com/us/blog/the-baby-scientist/201907/why-children-repetition-and-how-it-helps-them-learn.

136. Simple Puzzles

1. Team Lovevery, "Puzzling over Puzzles—What the Progression Looks Like," Lovevery, last modified July 15, 2022, https://lovevery.com/community/blog/child-development/puzzling-over-puzzles-what-the-progression-looks-like/.

137. Sippy Cups

1. "Sippy Cup," Wikipedia Foundation, last modified May 25, 2025, https://en.wikipedia.org/wiki/Sippy_cup.

138. Baby Talk

1. Lauren Lowry, "Baby Babble: A Stepping Stone to Words," The Hanen Centre | Speech and Language Development for Children, February 13, 2017, https://www.hanen.org/Helpful-Info/Articles/Baby-Babble--A-Stepping-Stone-to-Words.aspx.

139. Bringing Toys

1. Jen Lumanian, "An Age-by-Age Guide to Teaching Your Child to Share," July 25, 2018, https://yourparentingmojo.com/sharing/.

140. Going for a Cruise

1. "Cruising: Preparing Baby for First Independent Steps," BabySparks, last modified August 10, 2017, https://babysparks.com/2017/08/10/cruising-preparing-baby-for-first-independent-steps/.

141. Calming Down by Myself

1. "Cruising: Preparing Baby for First Independent Steps," BabySparks, last modified August 10, 2017, https://babysparks.com/2017/08/10/cruising-preparing-baby-for-first-independent-steps/.

142. Come Here

1. "70 Funny Parents Quotes That Sum Up Parenting to a Tee," Rookie Moms, accessed September11, 2022, https://www.rookiemoms.com/funny-parenting-quotes/.

143. Turning On the TV

1. Cat Bowen, "Here's Why Your Baby Is Straight-Up *Obsessed* with Your Remote,"

Romper, May 28, 2019, https://www.romper.com/p/why-do-babies-love-remote-controls-their-electronic-obsession-isnt-too-hard-to-understand-17924440.

144. Hold My Hand

1. Gwen DeWar, PhD, "When Do Babies Start Walking, and How Does It Develop? (An Illustrated Guide)," PARENTING SCIENCE, last modified August 3, 2022, https://parentingscience.com/when-do-babies-start-walking/.

145. Going to the Store

1. "15 Tips for Parenting in Public," Peaceful Parenting, accessed September 15, 2022, https://www.ahaparenting.com/read/discipline-in-public-tips.

146. Copying Words

1. "A Quote by Reba McEntire," Goodreads accessed September 15, 2022. https://www.goodreads.com/quotes/80552-watch-what-you-say-and-do-because-little-eyes-are.

147. Are You Listening?

1. Focustherapy, "When a Child Doesn't Respond to Their Name: Speech-Language Pathologist Insights," the *Focus* blog, last modified September 6, 2022, https://focusflorida.com/speech-therapy/when-a-child-doesnt-respond-to-their-name-speech-language-pathologist-insights/.

148. Mama!

1. Cori, "Mom Burnout: Symptoms of Mom Burnout & Strategies for Being Happier," The Pragmatic Parent, last modified July 30, 2020, https://www.thepragmaticparent.com/7-ways-cure-mom-burnout/.

149. Directing Your Hand

1. "Reading Books to Babies," Nemours Kidhealth, accessed September15,2022, https://kidhealth.org/en/parents/reading-babies.html.

150. Favorite Toys

1. Rogers, "When Do Babies Start Playing with Toys?" What to Expect.

151. STANDING ALONE

1. "Take a Stand! How to Help Baby Stand on Their Own," Pathways.org.

152. SHOWING FEAR

1. Rebecca Parlakian, "Childhood Fears," ZERO to THREE, October 11, 2019, https://www.zerotothree.org/resource/childhood-fears/.

153. BEWARE BLUE LIGHT

1. Jay Vera Summer, "How Blue Light Affects Kids' Sleep," Sleep Foundation, last modified July 23, 2025, https://www.sleepfoundation.org/children-and-sleep/how-blue-light-affects-kids-sleep.

154. STRIKE UP THE BAND

1. First Word Projects, "Baby and Toddler Milestones: 16 Actions with Objects by 16 Months," Reading Rockets.

155. TRYING TO SING

1. Ben Millam "How to Raise Musical Children: Birth to Age 5," the *Benjamin Millam* blog, last modified January 13, 2021, https://benjaminmillam.com/music-education/how-to-stimulate-your-childs-musical-mind-birth-to-age-5/.

156. WHERE'S YOUR HEAD?

1. Jennifer Kelly Geddes, "Learning How to Identify Body Parts," What to Expect, last modified March 3, 2015, https://www.whattoexpect.com/toddler/toddler-growth-and-development/learning-body-parts.aspx.

157. PICK ME UP

1. Anticipatory Adjustments to Being Picked Up in Infancy," PubMed Central (PMC), accessed September 18, 2022, https://www.ncbi.nlm.nih.gov/pmc/articles/PMC3688725/.

158. RESISTING

1. Sheryl Sandberg, "Trying to Do It All and Expecting That It All Can Be Done Exactly Right Is a Recipe for Disappointment ..." | 16 Inspirational, Funny and Refreshingly Honest Working Mom Quotes | Chaos & Quiet," Pinterest, Last modified October 31, 2018, https://www.pinterest.com/pin/271130840056755986/.

159. FLIPPING PAGES

1. “How Books Develop Fine Motor Skills,” BabySparks, last modified March 9, 2020, https://babysparks.com/2020/03/09/how-books-develop-fine-motor-skills/.

160. BABY IS WALKING

1. “Delay in Walking,” Patient | Professional Articles | Paediatrics | Delay in Walking, last modified April 26, 2019, https://patient.info/doctor/delay-in-walking.

www.ingramcontent.com/pod-product-compliance
Lightning Source LLC
Chambersburg PA
CBHW060403130626
46555CB00005B/1985

* 9 7 9 8 9 9 9 8 9 9 9 0 3 *